The Life Reset

Reclaim Your Time, Boost Your Energy and Rediscover Yourself

Leanne Barriball

The Life Reset- Reclaim Your Time, Boost Your Energy and Rediscover Yourself

All views expressed in this publication are the authors own, through her own personal experiences. They are not to be reprinted or shared without prior consent of the author.

Where quoting about Neuroscience, Neuro-coaching this information has been obtained through Dr Shannon Irvine, who the author trained under to get a SINC Neuro-coaching Qualification. Any further information can be found on her website.

Copyright © 2025 Leanne Barriball
All Rights Reserved
ISBN:
Imprint: Independently published

Forward

Do you want to reclaim your time? boost your energy? Create the life you have always wanted? This book will help you to start the process.

Leanne's second book takes you on a learning trip inside your own mind. You will find yourself realising that you are not alone when you feel overwhelmed. You will learn new strategies that will bring you to a point where you are loving and enjoying your daily life. By the end of the book, you will feel ready to embrace your new self and life.

Edited with love by SJBB

Dedication

This book is dedicated to my lovely mum who is pictured here hanging out my washing as my physical health has taken a different turn this year. I will be forever grateful that you were chosen to be my mum, especially as I know I am not an easy daughter to live with sometimes, but I get on my high horse with the best intentions to see us all thriving not just surviving as a family.

Thank you for your time, patience and love for us all you really do mean the world to us.

Ps Mum please read this book and do the steps you deserve some you time as well

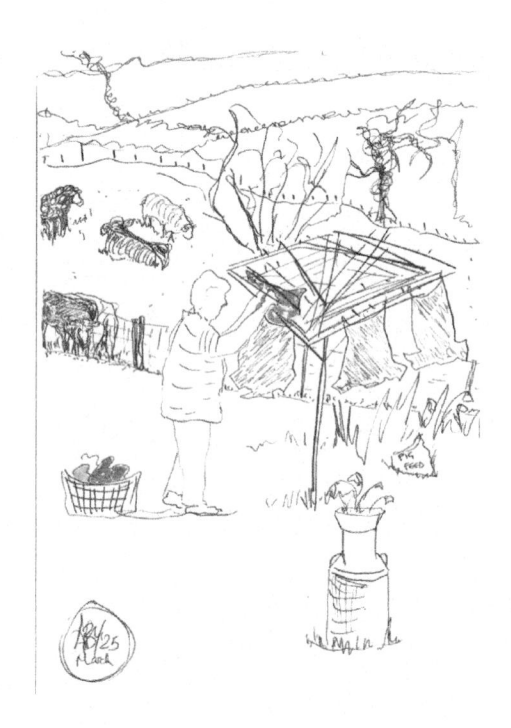

CONTENTS

Introduction

Chapter 1- Rewiring from overwhelm

Chapter 2- Breaking the busy cycle

Chapter 3- Getting the brain unstuck

Chapter 4- Reframing our thoughts

Chapter 5- Choosing a different future

Chapter6- Fear has the same chemicals as excitement

Chapter 7- Capturing thoughts before they catch you

Chapter 8- Overcoming- I'm not good enough cycle

Chapter 9 – Breaking free from perfectionism

Chapter 10- Coaching versus counselling

Chapter 11- Restoring your energy and identity

Chapter 12- Learning to be a better role model

Chapter 13-You try everything and nothing sticks

Chapter 14- What is your why?

Chapter 15- Your vision for the 2.0 version of you

Chapter 16- Building healthy boundaries

Chapter 17- The challenges you may face

Chapter 18- Choose your village wisely

Chapter 19- Failure is the key to success

Chapter 20- Slowing down to speed up

Conclusion

Appendix 1- Vision Sparks

Appendix 2-Brain blocks

Appendix 3- Emotions and Where in the Body

INTRODUCTION

Hey friend! I am so grateful that you are here with me on this journey. I created this book because I used to feel that it was impossible to do everything that I wanted to do in life. To be a mum, to be healthy and happy, to run a business as a Tropic Ambassador, and to start a new business! To do all the things I absolutely adore doing with my friends and family, like having cups, of tea BBQs and genuinely living a good life.

In the quest to discover how I could make what I felt impossible, possible, I created the contents of this book to share with you. I want you to see that it is possible to look after your health, be a great mum, and do all the things that you feel like you want to do in life. Whether that's being super mum, having a business, art, music, or teaching. Anything that you feel that you would love to do can become possible.

In this book, I am going to show you how I discovered that we can do it all. How we can put our own health first, whilst still honouring our family by being present, and making strategic steps towards making your dreams come true, which for many of us is for everyone in our family to be happy and healthy.

A little about me if you haven't already read my first book "Farming Broke Me But I Keep Fighting" which is available on Amazon.

I am a farmer's daughter who lives on the Devon and Cornwall Border (Devon side) of the UK. I was born into our farming business, which is a very interesting and sometimes complicated place to be born, primarily because us farmers tend to keep following in footsteps which aren't always good for us.

As is the saying, *"the definition of insanity is keep repeating the same things and expecting different results"*.

I have a daughter, Hayley, who was born in 2014, and she is home educated. The home-education side of life started because I needed to help and support her with her mental and emotional health. Hayley did go to school, but we decided to take her out when she couldn't cope anymore. This change in education meant that a lot of things had to change in our daily life, especially in my life, it took a while to adjust. I had to change how I was using my time, to give enough of it to ensuring Hayley had all the skills she needs to succeed in the world.

I also had a deep desire to start and run my own coaching business, helping women to approach their own lives in the same manner as I have been doing. I have become the person I needed at the beginning of this journey to help others. I wanted to be able to do all the things I wanted to do, as well as be present with Hayley, so that she feels loved, worthy and safe all the time without getting burnt out, this was the tricky bit!

To feel loved, worthy and safe, are the 3 key brain-based fundamentals that every human needs to become stable and capable adults. Most of these are set in the first 3-5 years of life. If things go wrong then and trauma is experienced it can take a little time to work things through, but anything is possible and things can change, as I found out with my Hayley girl.

In this book, I want you to learn how to claim back your time, rather than letting it run away from you. I want you to feel fulfilled and good about yourself, and above all to be healthy from the inside out, in order for you to thrive not just survive. I will show you that when you prioritise slowing things down and resting, you not only become more organised, but you will have a lot more energy and you may just find yourself enjoying the little things in life again. Let's face it, feeling like super mum and having more energy is a big bonus!

By learning to slow your life down, going so slow at times you actually stop, which I have done many times. When you reach this place of stopping, you can truly trust that the next steps are going to be amazing. Your brain slowing down for you to be able to speed up, is essentially allowing your thinking to level up.

Anyone reading this that resonates with an ADHD neurotype this is for you too, believe it or not.

I am also going to show you how important it is to find out what your purpose is beyond motherhood, because one day when you're not needed as much anymore as a mum its good for you to have something for you to get into that's yours.

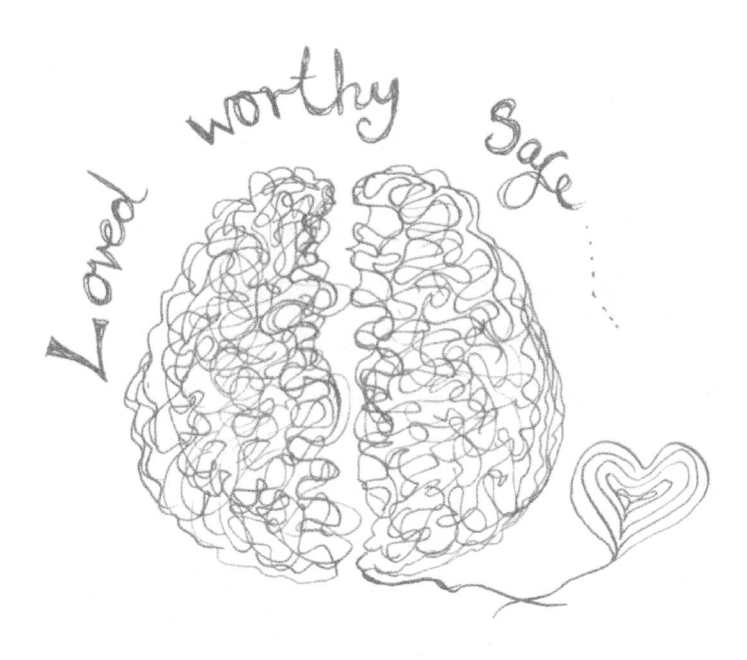

Have you considered this before? What is it you are good at? What would you like to do in the future? I believe that every single person has a reason to be here, and we each need to step into this purpose to help each other. The biggest challenge we have is connecting to our inner selves and trusting our intuition enough to be able to know what our heart really longs to do.

Ultimately though, we humans are here to help one another. For some of us, it may be to help 1 person, others it maybe 5 people, 1000 or even millions! Life can be difficult I know what it feels like to not know or believe that you're here for any reason at all, that you're just existing in what seems like a chaotic and frightening world, unsure what the future holds. Fear is real but you don't have to let it win.

By focusing in on managing your time more effectively, getting rid of the busy brain, and even learning to sleep better, you will create more energy, and have more of a desire to discover what your purpose is. You will then be able to live a life that you love living, and can be proud of being your best self.

I am going to show you how you can manage your time in such a way that you are literally choosing what you do, hour by hour, or minute by minute if you want to. And to do it in such a way that it becomes automatic just like brushing your teeth, so you don't even have to consciously think about it, it just happens. This happens by simply learning to change how you think.

This will unlock more energy to spend with your kids, to consider things to do to take care of your health and even go dancing if that's your thing. Children want our time and undivided attention; they don't need material things; they need us present and enjoying them. We only have them for a short time before they move onto their own lives. If our attention is constantly drifting off and we can't focus on anything, it makes everyone feel rubbish in the end and this doesn't have to happen anymore.

I am going to teach you how you can start to think differently to create a life that you may feel is impossible right now, but it doesn't have to stay that way. It all starts with your thoughts, and what you are thinking for 90 percent of your time. This is how your brain makes decisions and then acts creating the results you want or for most of us the ones we don't want.

CHAPTER 1- REWIRING FROM OVERWHELM

If you are still here, then that means something in what I have said has piqued your interest. I want to share with you a couple of situations where I have personally used the strategies in this book. I am completely practicing what I preach in this regard, I am a true believer in going through the process myself because transformed people, transform people.

I became a mum to a beautiful, bouncing baby girl. The challenge I had was that I completely lost my physical health, and it took me two and a half years to be able to walk without crutches again. It was such a challenging time for me, my mental and emotional health went down the drain, I was a mess at the time when I wanted to be enjoying being a new mum, and soak up the baby snuggles.

To help myself get out of the dark pit I was in, I joined a company called Tropic, as an ambassador and started selling their skin care. I absolutely loved it, and this was the beginning of my self care journey because the 5 minutes I spent either end of the day giving myself a facial, became a time I started enjoying and I had a desire to do even more things to help me to feel better inside and out.

The problem was, I really struggled to keep on top of the daily tasks, like cleaning, cooking, washing and taking care of my toddler. At the time it was a daily battle, the overwhelm was real and I now know that it was all in my head. My mind was a battlefield!

I was exhausted all the time trying to do all the things I needed to do. Having a child to look after does that to us and is especially difficult if you don't know how to spend time on yourself before you have the baby.

This is a life lesson anyone reading this who isn't a mum yet!

My mind was literally wired to be in chaos, made worse by all the fears, guilt and shame which we can have as mums as well just trying to keep our kids alive. Overwhelm is a mechanism our brain uses to keep us safe, when it thinks that something terrible is happening based on what thoughts we have to situations.

This is why different people can react to the same situation in a different way. We all have different thought processes that trigger off, and this creates a physical reaction in the body under the name of e-motions. Or Energy in motion.

Overwhelm is a warning sign that something needs to be changed. That you don't feel safe, loved or worthy.

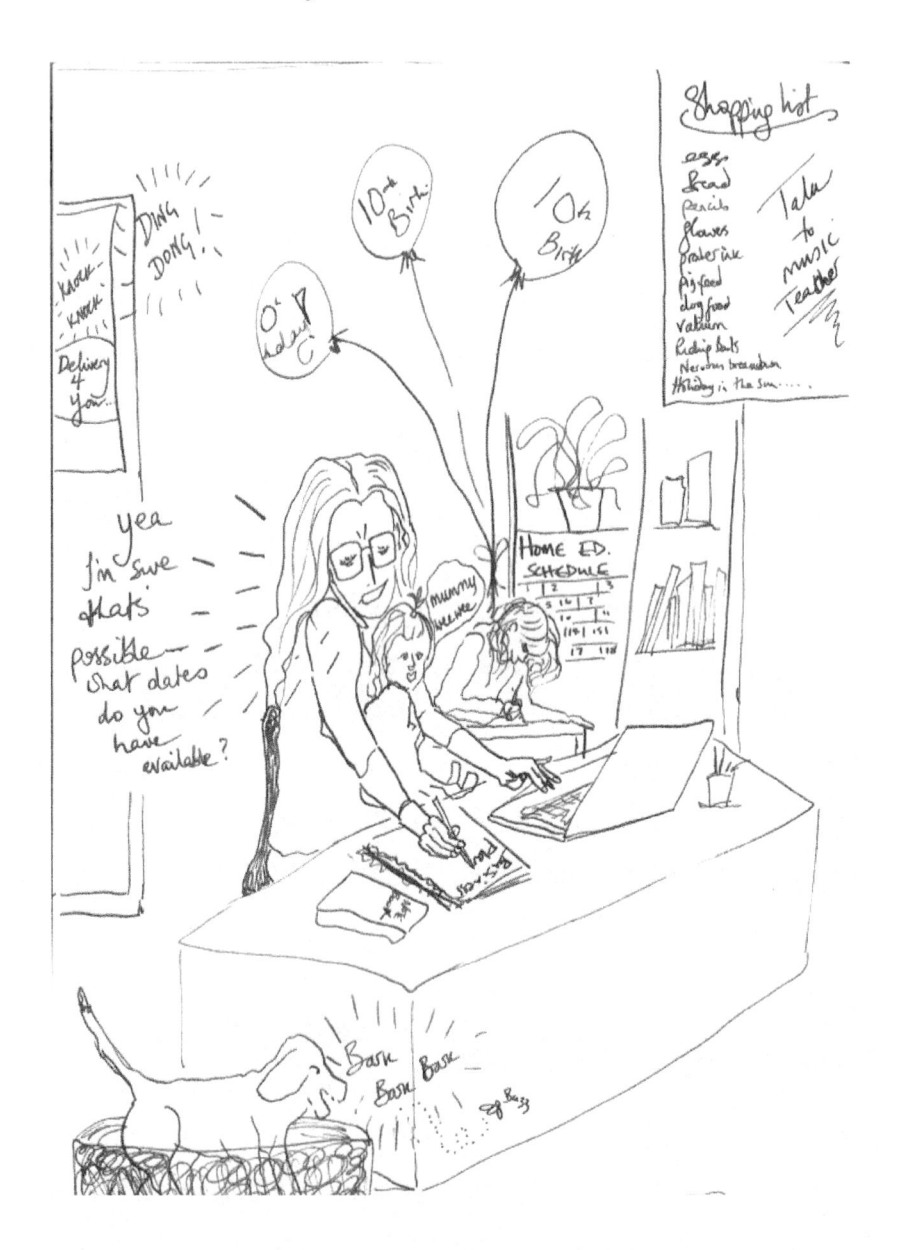

One day I was listening to a podcast by Dr Caroline Leaf, she was talking about neuroplasticity and the ability we have to rewire our thoughts, that we were originally designed to operate in love not fear, and this is what can give us many mental and emotional health problems. The fear can often be our own thoughts sabotaging us, keeping us so busy we just stumble through life hoping one day for a breakthrough, that may never come unless you become aware these things are happening, you have the choice to change things.

Try this

Take a pen and paper and set a timer for 20 minutes. In those 20 minutes try (try being the operative word) and catch all the thoughts you can hear going through your mind. I learnt a big lesson with this exercise.

In those 20 minutes I wrote down the biggest mess of thoughts that I ever did read! It was so bad in fact I had to burn it. I wish I hadn't now because it would show me how far I have come. It was in that moment I realised that my mind was my problem, it was just far too busy all the time, thinking about things I didn't even need to think about. My own brain was making me exhausted and inefficient.

Back then when I didn't know any better, I used to think it was the brain, but it is the subconscious mind where our thoughts will, and emotions are. It's the part of the brain that gives instructions to your body automatically, it tells you to breathe, blink, move your arms and it also controls what you do daily. Imagine what happens if your subconscious mind has not been trained in such a way to make life easier, that in fact it could be making your life harder. Self-sabotage, procrastination, perfectionism all learnt behaviours which are coming from the instructions within your subconscious mind.

I thought I had lost my physical health first whilst I was pregnant, but now I know it was my mental and emotional health that caused my physical health break down. I was not taking care of my body in anyway. I slept badly, I ate badly, and I worked all hours God sent, because my worth was in doing not being, until I couldn't work anymore, and I became a baby oven. It sounds dramatic but I had been set up by my own thoughts to destroy myself. Which sounds mad when you hear it like that, but it is the truth. I could not show myself love, I did not feel worthy, and I never felt safe (because I never slept well) and to stop these feelings I kept myself really busy all the time, so I didn't have to deal with it. This was not a good choice on my part.

You may ask "well where do these thoughts come from?" As babies we are all born as a clean sheet. I was not born with 60,000 thoughts rushing around my mind. These thoughts can come from generational habits which get passed down through families and cultures. Children learn from role models, so whoever the role models are in a child's life, they are the ones they copy. The good, the bad, and the downright ugly.

Children need to be shown healthy behaviours from their role models. If they have not been shown healthy ways to take care of themselves mentally and emotionally, then it goes without saying the child will pick up the same habits. This is not just relevant to parents now; this could go back generations.

There is a whole heap of thoughts I have had to face up to in my mind, that have been passed down to me from at least 5 generations of our farming family. I have observed that every generation this has caused a little more damage as its moved down, creating a complete mess of inherited thoughts and behaviours when it came to me, and the generations I still live with. When I realised this was even a thing, I decided to stop it, so that these negative thoughts and beliefs could no longer operate in me or my family. This work has been life changing.

In 2020, I discovered a way that I could rewire my brain, retrain it, and become more disciplined so I could do the daily stuff that needed to be done by making it automatic, but also be a present mum who knew exactly what it is her daughter needed every day. I used to write down everything that was taking up my time, whether it was my business, the farm, my health, the cleaning or the cooking, I just wrote it down. I thought "how can I change this? What do I want my time to look like?" and I started to plan where I could ultimately create order and automate the so called boring but necessary things of life, like cleaning. Whilst finding space for the things I wanted to do, like writing books.

As a person who is self-diagnosed with ADHD, I can say that there are a lot of tasks that need to be done where we do not have enough dopamine to do them. This is because the steps can be missing subconsciously. Which means the simplest tasks can get on top of us and create overwhelm. But the brain can be retrained and this is what makes this work exciting.

This is just a snippet of what I have done, to enable myself to stop wasting precious time and I am now able to help others do the same, and that ultimately, is the purpose of this book.

Client Testimonies

Client 1 has two young boys; she works part time as a teacher and her husband is a farmer. She always felt tired and would get bouts of depression where she struggled to get out of bed, and she felt everything was just too overwhelming. She also had to do the planning for her class, but all she wanted was to be more present for her own children. She could not see a way to do everything she needed to do, as a mum wife and teacher, let alone the things she wanted to do which was to spend quality connected time with her children.

As her coach I was able to help her see that she is in control of her thoughts and more importantly catch what they are. That she can think about what her ideal day would look like and then show this to her brain, (which is easier than you think). The brain then starts to create a new thought pattern or neural network, which in turn will prompt your brain to start giving you the steps, through your reticular activating system (RAC) that you need to be able to reach the goal of being more present, and lots less overwhelmed.

This helped give my client more energy and the feeling of satisfaction that she isn't missing out on her boys growing up.

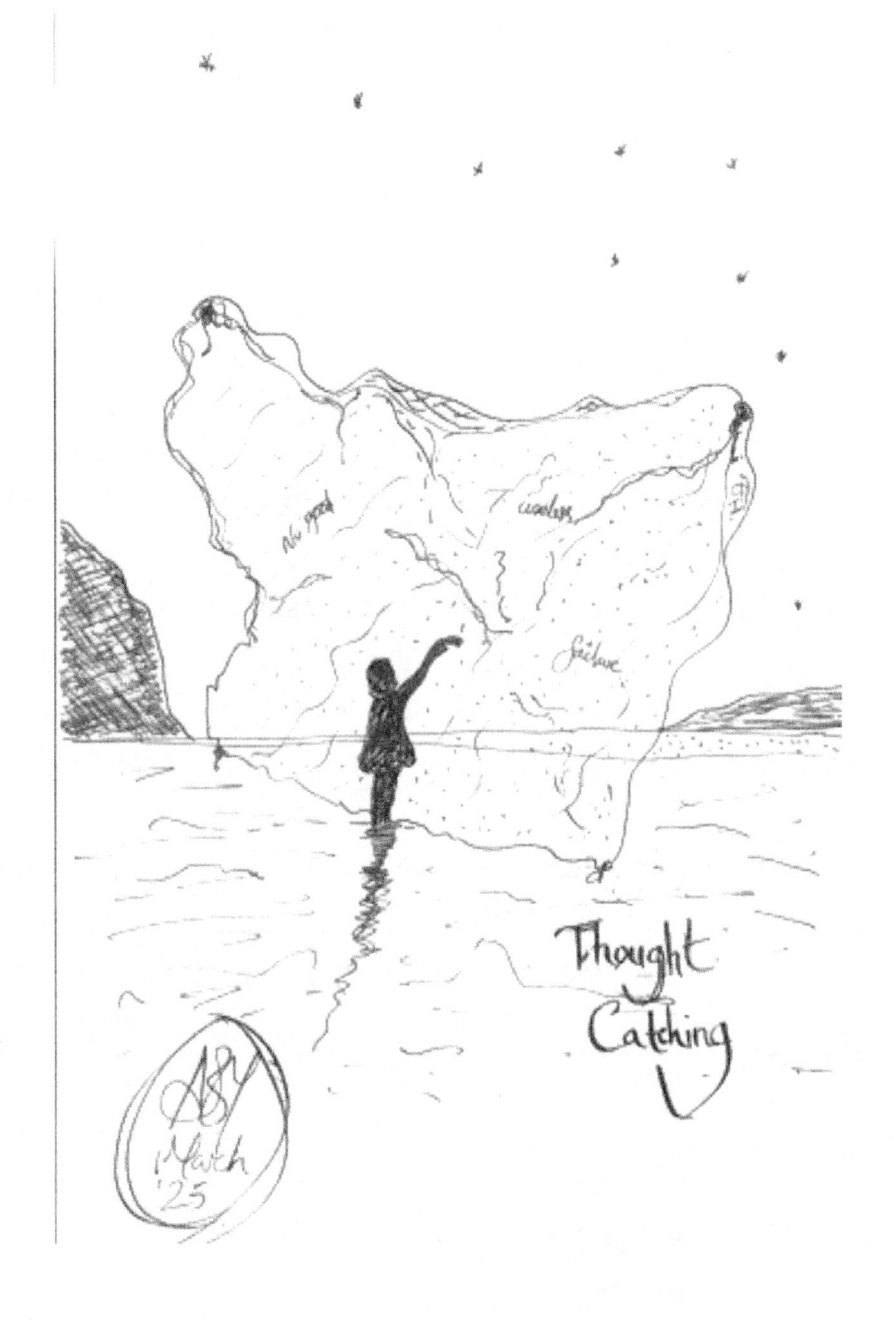

As I mentioned before 90 percent of the decisions we make daily, are made subconscious so automatic. Therefore, we have no idea we are making them. You know like when we eat a whole packet of biscuits and wondering how or why did I do that? These decisions are being made based on things we have learned through observation or repetition from the past. It only takes 67 repetitions to create a new thought process which isn't very many and is how we can become sublimely programmed by things, take adverts for example or even school if I am to get controversial.

This is how you can see whole families with similar ways of doing things because we learn them, the good things that will serve us in life and take us far, and of course the bad things that can become a problem eventually, and get you asking yourself "why can't I do things others seem to be able to?" This doesn't mean you are broken or a bad person it just means there is some faulty wiring in your brain, and it just needs rewiring, which we now know how to do.

The best bit is this goes for anything in life, from what you want your health to be like, how to manage your time which could be so well that you end up with spare time to do whatever you want.

I helped my client in the exact same way that I had helped myself as a mum with a brain that was too busy. I helped her to become more present with her boys, enabling her to do the job that she wanted to do, as well as keeping her house organised, and have time to do fun things as well. Ultimately there are days where she feels like a super mum, and we all need more of those days!

Client 2 who recently had a baby girl, was already running a coaching business teaching kids parkour, and trying to grow her business. She wanted to hire a new coach so that she could have time off when she had her baby. I helped her while she was pregnant, to get her business to a place of being able to run itself for her to have a break. Since having the baby, we have worked on how she can manage her time so she is still present with her daughter and able to work from home.

I have enabled her to think in such a way, that she is able to do all the things she wants to do, and all the things that she needs to do, for herself and her family. Our subconscious thoughts are driving our daily decisions and for many of us those thoughts are of being so busy we have become unproductive. Hopefully you can start to see that you have the power to change that.

This is what makes what I do so exciting, because it means the possibilities are limitless, there is nothing stopping any of us to reach the goals we want to reach, other than our faulty thought patterns of course, which I have just told you, we can change.

And because I have been there and literally done what it is I hope and dream I can help you achieve, then it can happen quicker and easier for you. I have done the hardest bits for you, I have gone ahead, made the mistakes and worked out the short cuts.

Whether it's becoming healthier, mind, body, soul, starting a business, going to work and enjoying it, or knowing and feeling that your kids are happy and fully taken care of because you've been present with them, and you know the exact things they need to thrive. I encourage you to embark on this journey and start rewiring your overwhelmed brain.

CHAPTER 2- BREAKING THE BUSY CYCLE

I have shared with you a little bit about myself and why I have written this book, I have shared a little bit about some of my clients and how I have been able to help them by implementing what I'm teaching you in this book.

I want to dive a little deeper into how I have helped myself get the results that I wanted. For me that meant I wanted to be a fantastic mum, keeping on top of household chores and have things organised and tidy. I wanted to spend time with my friends and family and be there if they needed me which is a big thing in today's world. I was also aware we were running our farming business, and I wanted that farming business to start thriving and to ultimately look after itself.

That things would become easier, and the farm would start taking care of us, rather than us having to take care of it, which is a huge mindset shift in itself if you are a farmer or know one. Huge changes have had to be made for us to get some structure, and to start running it as a sustainable business rather than a lifestyle, that had become unhealthy, because our busy thought life was making things unproductive, hard work and exhausting.

I also had this burning passion to help other mums who have got the same problems I had when I first had Hayley. In the beginning I just thought "I'm never going to be able to do all of this, something is always going to have to give, it's always going to cost something".

Up until that point, the cost of me believing it was all about doing doing doing, and being super busy was my health. Then when I became a mum, everything shifted, and it all became about Hayley rather than me, working hard to earn money all the time, and things got even worse. I felt like my brain was spinning all the time and I was getting nowhere. I remember realising one day that I thought I was doing loads of things in a day, but it was all in my head. There was no outward actions being taken because my brain was just too busy trying to work out what was going on, made worse by my terrible sleeping habits, which was not helping anything.

How could I do it all? how could I be present for my daughter? whilst doing all these other things that I love doing and fulfil me? Thankfully the answer was within the realms of neuroscience and my own neural pathways (thoughts).

I love being busy, I love helping people, I love being the person that someone comes to and says, "are you able to help me with this?" But I have had to learn to say no. I have had to learn to put my boundaries in place, and structure my life in such a way that I don't feel so exhausted any more. The more time I spend on myself and taking care of me, the more time I actually end up having for the people I love. If only I knew this before becoming a mum.

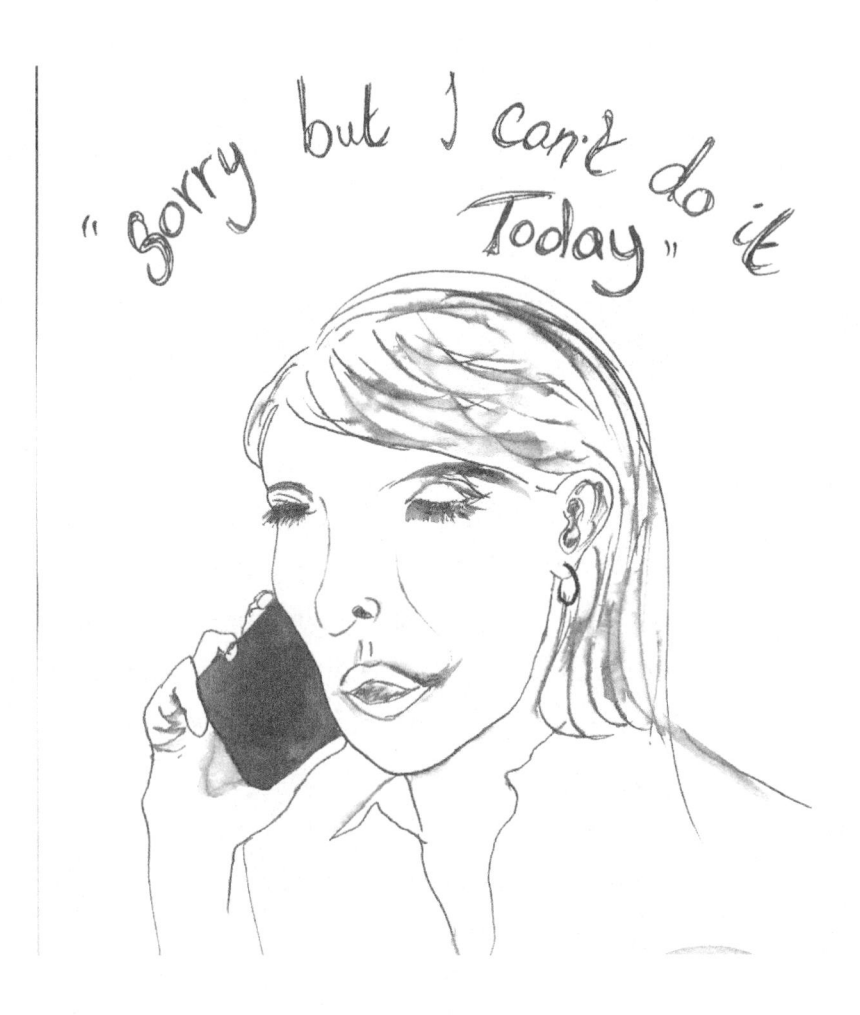

Whilst on the journey of discovering how I was going to do this, I realised that my most powerful asset is my own brain. I have known for a long time that I have an incredible brain. I have one of those brains that can learn and take in information that it needs and churn out information to teach and inspire others.

I'm a very logical thinker, I'm a deep thinker and I'm a problem solver. My greatest asset was sitting on top of my shoulders. The challenge I have had was that I was so stressed out, my body was addicted to cortisol and was always in fight or flight mode. Even today I am still challenged by too much cortisol being released because my body believed it needed it all the time to survive when the opposite is true. Too much cortisol burns us out, especially us ladies with our delicate hormones.

My brain believed that to be able to function, I needed to be stressed out to the max all the time, you could say it was running on negative energy not positive. Whilst on this journey (I am still on that journey), I have realised, "hang on a minute! I don't have to keep being this way anymore. If I want to be less stressed, then I get to choose to design a life that is calm, peaceful and full of joy more than be complete chaos and something I want to or need to escape from.

As I mentioned before, our thoughts are different to our brain. Our thoughts come from the subconscious mind. The subconscious is a part of us which is very cleverly designed to help us conserve energy. It works that when we repeatedly think something after 67 repetitions, it goes into our subconscious to help us stop using too much energy on that particular thought. The challenge we have if left unchecked is this very system can be used negatively with negative thoughts sucking out our energy rather than creating more.

Can you see that this is great for things like brushing our teeth and getting dressed which we need to do, however its dangerous if we are surrounded by negativity or hearing and seeing things that become our thoughts later down the line. Imagine how many thoughts your subconscious mind is holding, how many of them do you think are helping you with your daily actions? or are they keeping you wanting to stay in bed because it is so much safer there!

Through the help of neuroscience and the amazing people who are looking into how the brain works, I have learnt that our brains, or my brain, has been wired to burn itself out, and not to look after my health. My own brain was making decisions to finish me off early or I would end up having a hard time in my later years because I have burned my body out now.

We are burning ourselves out ladies. And of course, a large part of this is because we are living through a completely different age and time than our parents and don't we know it. We need to parent differently because the world we were brought up in is no longer the same.

A lot of the thoughts I had in my head were hatred towards myself. I didn't think I was worthy unless I was doing certain things. A big issue I had attached to lots of different thoughts was, I didn't feel safe a lot of the time. I think this feeling arose from a multitude of things from childhood through to my teens, and it doesn't have to be "big" situations, you must remember it can be as little as your guinea pig running away and thinking you had lost it forever, finding it and then it dies of the stress, the next day. That was a hard day for me, because my in-development brain which is every brain under the age of 22-24 could not comprehend it. Which is why subject to whatever you believe, children need situations explained to them, even ones we think are trivial.

Children are not as resilient as we have been led to believe, which is why we see so many struggling. They need the help of an adult with a fully developed brain, namely the prefrontal cortex to help them make sense of things.

The thoughts I am talking about you having in this book don't need to have come from your parents even. You may have had lovely parents who loved you so much, however they didn't have the depth of knowledge we now do around trauma.

I can remember the first person to die in my family was my great grandad, I was maybe 4 or 5. I remember my mum saying, "grandad has died at the hospital and isn't coming back". I remember lying in my bed and crying and not understanding what had happened, but little me didn't go and say anything because what was there to say? I wonder however if maybe my behaviour changed, I became a bit more "naughty" or 'whiny", because I have seen this in my daughter when she is processing grief and trauma. It is her behaviour that changes.

When children don't have the words to express their feelings, their feelings become motions E-motions energy in motion. Which is why if you have a child who is a "difficult" child then this needs to be considered because the slightest changes can upset them.

We are fighting an invisible battle in our minds, and if we aren't aware of it then this is what is catching us all out, making us feel depressed, anxious and stressed.

The Three Key Components to a Balanced Life

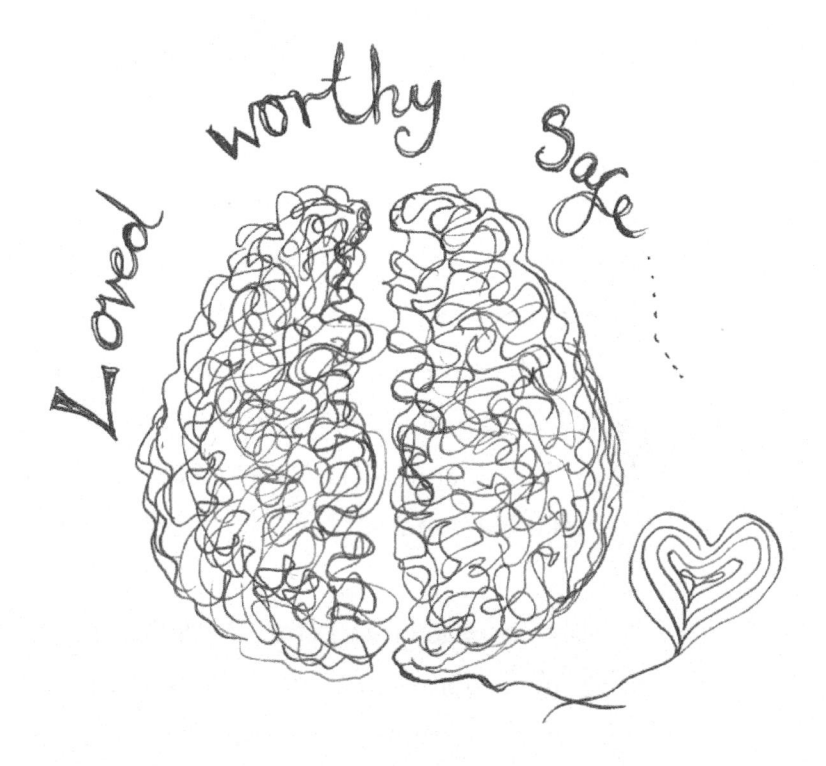

Now, this is a fascinating fact about training your brain, as I mentioned earlier, there is a part of the brain called the Reticular Activating System (RAS), it filters out irrelevant information and helps you to focus on what it thinks you need at that time, based on what you are telling it. For example, if you have ever considered getting a new car, suddenly you start to see that same car you are looking at everywhere. They have always been there it's just you notice now. The RAS can even get as specific as getting you to pick up a book off a shelf and finding the answer to your question inside, without reading the whole book! Which I personally think is really cool!

Lets put this into a real time situation which could help you out today! If you have the thought or even say the words " I am busy, or I am too busy, or I don't have time" then your (RAS) will be looking for all the reasons to make this the truth, and you wont get things done.

If however, you change the wording of these thoughts to "I have more than enough time today to do what I need to do" or "there is enough time today to get all my tasks done" your RAS will start looking for the steps you need to do to be productive and get things done.

How helpful would that be to you?

CHAPTER 3- GETTING THE BRAIN UNSTUCK

Now I have wired my brain to think in this new way, with the power of the reticular actuating system, it now looks for the people, the evidence, and situations that I need to make sure that the goals I have set myself are being met, and this works for anything, health, business and even relationships. Every step I need to take and decision I need to make comes from the amazing piece of equipment that is sitting on my shoulders called my brain! I used to think it was broken with its negativity bias, but all I needed to do was tap into it and start listening to harness my truest potential, which was there all along.

For my client who is a farmer's wife and has two young boys, whilst working with her, we discovered multiple situations where she had become stuck in her thought processes. Becoming stuck in a thought process, or you may be more familiar with the term "comfort zone" is just our brain trying to keep us safe with the information it has already.

When we start to rewire our thoughts though it can take a little time for our brain to work out that its ok, the new directions we are showing it are what we want to work towards, and this is when having a coach is key to get a full transformation and hit your goals quickly.

Our faulty thought patterns which may have served us well up to this point, if your alive reading this your brain has kept you safe. However, if you really check in with yourself are you really stressed all the time, exhausted, feeling like you are going around in circles? Your faulty thought patterns could be causing cortisol to release all the time and therefore creating an addiction to cortisol. Cortisol addiction is real, and it is what can be making us so tired, because it affects our adrenal glands, hormones and all our organs to be honest.

The next thing that happens is the body needs more energy to sustain the cortisol rushing through our veins, so it sends a signal for more food, and can you guess the food your body wants the most? I bet you can! the food with the highest energy to be released in the quickest time. You guessed it sugary foods, carb heavy foods, the ones that in your mind you think "I shouldn't eat this" but right then the need is too great and you cant over ride it, your body needs the energy to fight the imaginary war unstuck in your head.

The feeling of needing to eat the food is overwhelming then when you eat the food, you feel guilty, because everyone says not to eat these things.

(More to come in my next book about this topic)

We are then stuck in a cycle of being stressed, eating unhealthy food, and all because we have ultimately created or allowed our thought life to take over and create the stress, because the world is busy and we believe we need to be as well.

In farming we are very driven by this mentality. We work 365 days a year, seven days a week. We don't take holidays, we don't do bank holidays, we might have Christmas day off if we're lucky. When you have been raised in the farming way of life, you have been brought up to believe that the only way you fit in this world, is if you are working those hours. That you're not allowed a holiday because people will think you are lazy or something.

You believe you are getting judged and that someone is going to call in one day and catch you out, but it's not true. Who is the person who you believe is going to come in and catch you on the sofa resting at 4pm and say something derogatory? The reality is no one, and if they think it, that's their problem.

This mindset is burning us out, I was 24 and pregnant when that happened, and in this case, I do believe it's worse for us ladies because we have such a delicate balance of hormones. Leaving us susceptible to lower immune systems causing constant illnesses.

I am tired, stressed and I don't know what to do.

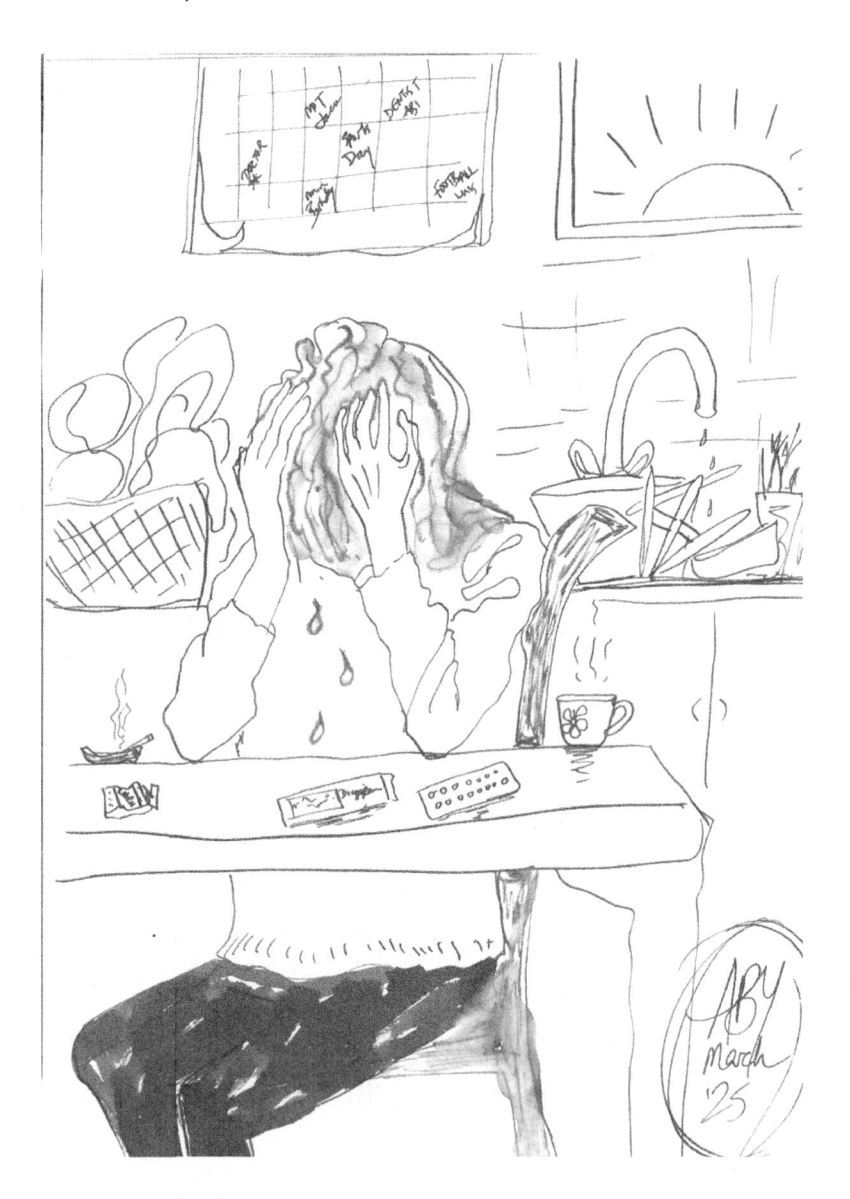

Scientists say our brain is thinking 60000 thoughts a day which is an exhausting figure in itself, and if those thoughts are more negative than positive because of our negativity bias which also happens in the human brain, and those thoughts are running 90 percent of your daily decisions and actions what do you think the end results are?

Look at your life through the new lens I have just shown you and you may just see a bit more of whats happening.

It can be so stressful! but I have enabled my clients to see around the mental blocks. We all have these thoughts that come up and say "no! you can't do that because………." This was a big issue for me. "No! you can't do that because you don't have enough time, you are too busy!". This all came from being called fat when I was around ten years old and believing that I wasn't good enough so I had to DO something about it.

I dread to think how many times that this thought has kept me from taking an opportunity to do something new.

There is also another faulty thought which I have helped my client and myself work through, "I am so lazy". Laziness can sometimes happen when the brain feels overwhelmed, that there is too much going on, so you literally zone out and you can't do anything. You think "Why!".

I have been through these kinds of situations where I feel stuck and I have no idea how to unstick myself. I was often blessed when it was right around my next call with my coaches, I would jump on a coaching call, (I am still being coached) and say "help I'm stuck!". My coaches who have also been certified in the SINC Neuro-coaching certification, are always able to help me to see the thought in my mind that is causing me to be stuck.

My second client who has just recently had a baby and is running a business, needed help with managing her time to be present with her daughter. She wanted to have a successful business, and bring in money so that she can give her daughter whatever she needs whenever she needs it. Working together we have been able to unstick her from her old thought patterns, which she had developed from childhood.

She believed that she had to do things in a set way, and if you didn't do things in a set way then you were not good enough, you were not honouring the family. These thoughts may have worked for her when she was a child, when she needed to do what she was being asked. But now as an adult it made it hard for her to push out and do new things.

Particularly when setting up a new business, as this takes a whole new set of skills! You must learn time management, and how to put in healthy boundaries so your business doesn't swamp you all the time. This is something us mums in business can struggle with because we really want to be successful and have more time freedom to spend with our family, which owning a business can create.

However, if we try running a business with a mindset that is set in working hard and long hours means you are worthy, you will never create time freedom in your business, where money just flows in every day and you don't have to work all the time or be the person that does everything, because your thoughts are working against you.

There many things that we know now, that many of us have no idea how to do in our lives, for me I feel sorry that school didn't teach me how to be financially stable to have a happy and home, not having to be the work force and do 9-5pm every day when really you just want to be with your children, and go to see Christmas plays and sports days when you want.

I didn't know I could be a stay-at-home mum whilst my daughter was little, and because we home educate her now whilst she is growing up as well. I am now starting to see the fruits of my thought process rewiring labours and be able to provide for our daughter in the best ways possible, because I dared for a moment to believe that things didn't have to keep being the way things were.

When I discovered Neuroscience and neuroplasticity it was the missing piece that I never knew I needed. They didn't know about this stuff 30 years ago but we know it now, and we owe it to our kids and ourselves to do something about it and make the changes. One thought at a time!! You don't have to tackle them all, just choose the thought that right now is at the forefront of your mind, I would hazard a guess it's around time and rewire it.

Our time is precious what are you doing with yours?

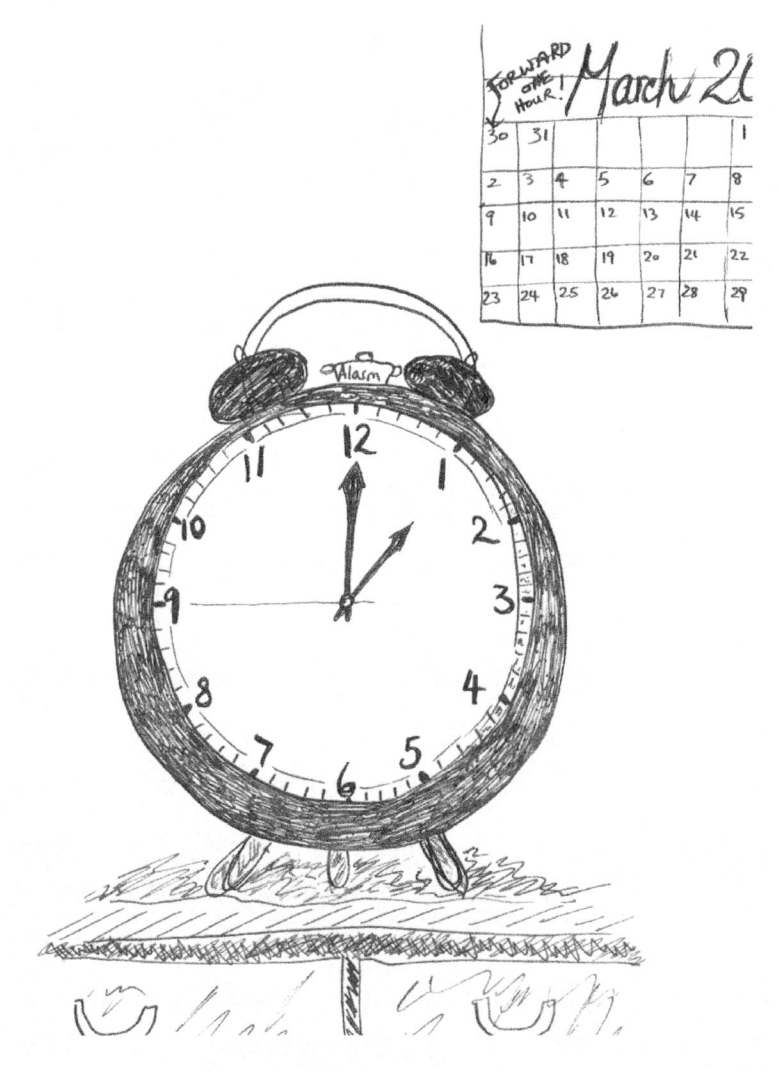

CHAPTER 4- REFRAMING OUR THOUGHTS

I went to school in the UK, and it did not teach me to manage my time well, particularly secondary school. It was like every hour, on the hour, you moved from one class to the next class, and looking back it was overwhelming. I think I did eleven different GCSEs, nothing that I could really get my teeth into and do a good job at. There were so many things to do that I was spreading myself thin, it was made even more difficult because I was a perfectionist. I took this way of doing things through my teens and into my twenties.

I was doing too many things and getting nowhere, so I basically had to go back and start again thinking about what I needed to think in order to create the life I wanted for me and my family.

This is now what I love to help other women to do, when a challenge comes up, they have a thought and have realised that this thought is keeping them from going forward. We are then able to talk it through, I help my client to see what they are thinking and then reframe it to what they want it to be, to move forward.

They can then break through and reach their goals. This is so exciting, because it means every single person on the planet, if they are willing to do the work, can think about what it is they want for their lives, and go get it! They can then create the life that they want, that they are truly proud of, and can look at their kids and think, "I am so glad I did this for them".

Since we have taken Hayley out of school in 2020, we have seen a huge positive difference in her mental and emotional health. She is growing up to be a confident, resilient, intelligent, kind and helpful young lady who is literally going to change the world around her. This is because even though I never imagined I would be home educating, I have been able to choose to invest more time into her and I have been able to create a clear vision for her life. Making a vision and focusing on helping her to get better has meant that all the provisions we have needed such as teachers, and finances have literally fallen into place, like puzzle pieces.

I have been able to see the exact steps we needed to take so she can start thriving. I believe that the decision we made back then although scary and I had no idea what would happen, was the right one for us and since then it is like my life has taken a direction for the better that I never knew was possible.

If you're a mum reading this today, and you want more than your current reality, then I encourage you to really think about what it is you need right now, and if it's something you have read in these pages then reach out.

I know for a fact that what I have learned about the brain and how we can reframe our thoughts and then rewire them to be automatic can work for you too. I have also realised that things haven't always turned out how I have wanted them to, but whilst I have been on this learning journey they have ended up better, and more aligned, helping me feel more in step with time than out of it. There is nothing more satisfying to me than to know and feel I am exactly the right place at the right time.

You know that feeling when something just works well, you met people in the right places on narrow roads (we have plenty in the southwest) or you think you are running late but you always get there on time, and calmly.

The truth is the answers to your own questions are hidden already in your own heart and mind and it just takes a reframed thought to get back on the right track.

CHAPTER 5- CHOOSING A DIFFERENT FUTURE

Years ago, I never really considered what my future would look like. I was so busy in the daily bump and grind it didn't cross my mind about what I wanted the future to be like even, I guess I believed it just happened, and I wasn't in control of anything. I always kind of knew I would be a mum, and that did happen. However, it doesn't look like how I was expecting it to look, and that's ok. Mainly because we have far more fun.

I always imagined that we would have two children close together, and in writing this book, we only have one child and she's coming up to ten years old. Although I had a vision for having 2 children, I don't think I was ever fully prepared for what it was going to be like being a mum to one child, especially with my health challenges that I am still healing from.

It sounds bizarre, but it comes with its own challenges, particularly when we needed to take her out of her school. I was met with the usual comments of "she will never be socialised" and even "you will never be able to do that". This seems to be the main thing that is said when you say you are home educating your child. But the truth is, she was not being social when she was in school, and she was not able to be social at home.

Whenever she would come home from school it would be a fight, whether it was on the pavement just outside or in the car. Then we would get home she would grab an iPad and stay glued to that thing all evening, her dad and I would try to engage, but it just was impossible, we were just met with lots of screaming and anger. Which sadly in the beginning was responded with shouting and anger, I have learnt a lot since then about how to control my own anger to help her.

Like many parents, we blamed ourselves. We said it was because we allowed her on technology, that we should have put better boundaries in place. However, it was not just that. This was our beautiful six-year-old girl telling us that she was in trouble, that she needed help, and instead of fighting it all the time, we made the changes. I have done the work on myself and have been blessed to make some different decisions which enabled us to have a much closer relationship and we enjoy spending time together. Hayley also has much healthier boundaries with technology which will set her up better for the future, when technology is going to be such a big part of our kids lives.

When I took her out of school, it was during Covid, which was Hayleys answer to prayer and made me brave, she was already out, so I knew that it was as good a time as any to send in the letter to deregister her. I remember thinking "how am I going to do it all?" but I knew in my heart I was going to have to work it out and make it happen. I was heavily involved (and still am) in our farming family business, I had my Tropic skincare business with lot of customers, and I was building a team of wonderful women. I was still on the journey improving my health and making myself feel better mentally, emotionally and physically.

I believed back then "I am never going be able to do everything!" I am going to have to give up everything now.

For three years my focus was, how I could build Hayley's confidence, help her to trust herself and trust me again and how she could become more resilient. Initially in a group environment, even with friends, Hayley would really struggle. One night it took her over an hour to come out and engage with friends of ours at a barbecue. All the other kids were running around, and she sat in the car, she just couldn't come out for fear. I have been able to give her the tools to work through her fears, because I work through mine.

We have worked on teaching her to take care of herself, when her mental health was at the lowest, her personal care really went downhill. She was not brushing her hair, or allowing me to brush it either, so it would get really knotty. I made it a thing that once a week for an hour and sometimes nearly 2 hours, I would sit and brush it for her, but it was very stressful at times.

Then it would get back to looking lovely again, and I would plait it ready for the following week. Hayley used to really struggle to have a shower or a bath, all the things that make us feel better. Sound familiar? I know adults who have this challenge, I have been one of them at times.

If we have not learnt self-care as a matter of necessity growing up it doesn't become a priority when we are grown up, and we choose not to do it, all the priorities of others come first leaving us spent of our energy.

Even though Hayley was so young, she was portraying what many adults are currently going through.
I have 100 percent been in that place where I have not wanted to get out of bed, have a shower, or not wanted to do anything. Even now, I occasionally dip back into those down days. However, when I discovered that I could choose to change this, a whole new world opened for me.

That world includes having friends and family around to help me when I need it. Just like Hayley needed me in her darkest times, I have needed the help of others as do you. The challenge many of us have is that we are too afraid to ask for help for fear that we are failing or being judged for needing the help. When the truth is the quicker we ask for the help, the quicker we get back on our feet again.

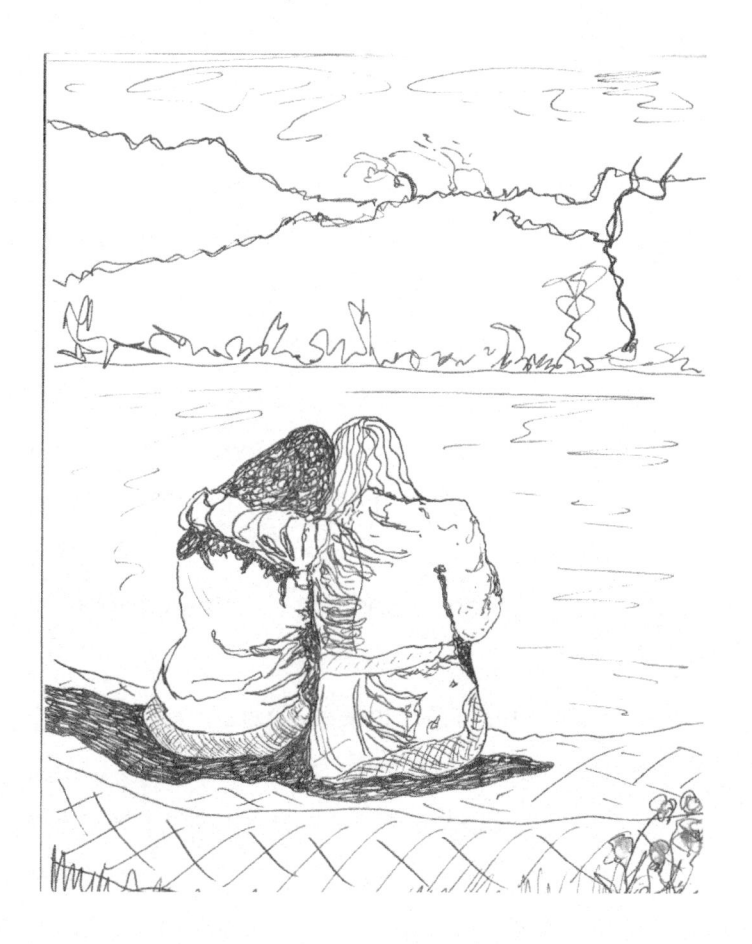

CHAPTER 6- FEAR HAS THE SAME CHEMICALS AS EXCITEMENT

I realised, "OK, so if I get to choose and I can rewire my thoughts to be able to run a more successful farming business, that will release some of my time". I hoped to get us to a place financially in the farming business that it would essentially run itself. I wanted to cut back my hours and not be doing the outside farming work so much, whilst Hayley and I found our home-educating feet.

This was not just about me, I wanted things to be simpler for my parents too, this was about honouring my mum and dad in this journey. They had their world turned upside down when we told them we were taking Hayley out of school, it was a new concept to them. When I was growing up very few kids were home educated, and in the last three years the numbers have grown dramatically. Even when we took Hayley out of school it was not as big as it is now.

Over the last three years we have made some important decisions about what we should do in our farming business, to make it more sustainable and so we can have a future in farming. A huge part of my heart is wanting farming to be an option in the future for Hayley and my brother's children.

Tropic was there for me when I had just had Hayley and my physical health was not great, but I still had to go through the process of letting go of what I had built. I had to let go of my team and customers, and I did a lot of things to put Tropic on the backburner, emotionally as well as mentally. It was scary to make that change, because I was wondering what I was stepping into, but I think a part of me was secretly excited.

I had to be a mum essentially 24 hours a day with no school time, and I had to also make sure that I was looking after myself, so I didn't burn out. I had not planned on being this mum, I assumed I was going to be like most mums in the UK and have a child in school from 5-16. Yet there was clearly another plan at play.

I remember in those early days, I would often ring up my father-in-law and just ask if I could go and sit in his house, light the fire and sit there for the whole afternoon. Have a cup of tea by myself and just be me. I would also often go to the car and just sit in a lay by alone. I had always thought I was an extrovert, but it turns out that there are times where I needed to be an introvert, where I needed my own space to refresh and recharge, so I could go back to my family a better version.

This has been something that has unfolded over time. I have learned to enjoy my own company, with a quieter mind. When I have had my alone time, I have more energy for when I need to be an extrovert, or deal with highly emotional situations with Hayley, which in the beginning there were many. When you think about time to yourself what do you tell yourself? "That you don't have time for that" "that you have too big of to do list to make time for you?" What thoughts pop up when you consider needing time to refresh and recharge however that looks?

I have realised on this journey that, "oh my goodness my brain is plastic, that Neuroplasticity is a thing, and I can really rewire my thoughts to create a better, happier more fulfilled life not just for me but for the rest of my family as well, because that's what we want isn't it? We want our families to be happy and healthy, and I am here to tell you that it starts with YOU being happy and healthy and full of energy.

If you are none of these things at the moment, then ask yourself why not? and start making plans to change it sooner rather than later. My main aim is to make sure that my health does not get so bad I become a bigger burden to my family than a help.

Fear is our biggest enemy, and the basis for nearly every negative thought that we have. Fear is a huge problem for all of us whether we know it or not, and fear can raise its ugly head in so many ways and this is how we are "triggered".

Fear is a powerful emotion, and it can get so overwhelming that it stops us from doing anything, especially when it comes to making changes. Many times I have had thoughts pop up that have tried to stop me changing our situation and I have been so afraid, literally I could wake up sweating. At the beginning of this process, I was having hundreds of negative sub-conscious thoughts a day which were not helping me to be successful, they would trigger an emotional response and this is what made me so exhausted.

I was shattered literally doing nothing physically. My brain on the other hand was constantly whizzing around. If anyone asked me if I was stressed, I would always respond with "No I am ok", when in reality I was so sub consciously stressed it had become the norm. My body was saying in many ways, we are exhausted I had constant stomach issues a knot in my tummy, I couldn't sleep properly, I would wake up shattered, I was heavily relying on carbs and sugar to get me through the day, but would still crash between 2-4pm needing a nap.

Looking back I can see I was wrecked but I had to work it out for myself. This is why when most women now explain their lives to me, and what their health is doing, and how they manage their time, I can see that they are tired, their face shows it, their body posture shows it, the way they are talking shows it. Ultimately, I have been there so I see it even more, and this enables me to get better and faster results for others.

This is the joy of being a coach because its these things that I help others to see, I help my clients to see what they are thinking, what they are feeling and most importantly how they need to think and believe to make changes to their thoughts now, to create a different future for themselves.

This isn't me telling you what to think either, this is all coming from within you. I show you what your brain is doing so you can then make the decisions on what to do with it. This is no hypnosis, or anything along those lines. This is me showing you what your own brain is up to.

CHAPTER 7- CAPTURING THOUGHTS BEFORE THEY CAPTURE YOU

The day when I knew I needed to deregister Hayley from school, I was so afraid, but I knew in my heart of hearts I needed to do it. I wrote the letter and sent it; I was so scared I thought "oh my goodness what have I done?" Then came the battle inside of me, I learned quickly that I needed to catch these thoughts else this was going to be a very stressful situation indeed.

I have written reams and reams of A4 lined note books, where I have caught my thoughts many of these being fears which brought in my fight or flight response, and in some ways stopped me from moving forwards. I realised that I was stressed so much of the time that I didn't know what it was like to not be stressed. The truth is how I was feeling, and acting was not how I wanted to feel or act.

There are times now when I am completely calm, and there are times when I am so stressed it is unreal. But I feel the difference now. I can say, "hang on a minute, why am I stressed? This is not what I want to be like", and one of the things I primed my brain to do was be more peaceful and less stressed so that my hair would stop turning grey!

I listened to a video once that suggested, if we get our body to the right place, the right equilibrium again, we could reverse grey hair. For three years I was waiting for my hair to appear, and then a few months ago, I sat there, and I picked up a hair that had fallen from my head, and there was it was a strand had been restored. It was brown from the root, so it was brown, grey brown. I knew then in that moment, that I was completely onto something, that I was able to reverse my stress and essentially the early ageing process, by capturing my thoughts that were based in fear, and stop me from becoming the woman who I desperately knew I didn't want to be.

Becoming the mum that I wanted to be. I wanted to be the fun mum, I wanted to be the extravagant mum who can dance and sing at the drop of a hat, literally burst into song in the middle of a kitchen. Okay, it's going to embarrass Hayley, but ultimately it would make her laugh, and that is what I have wanted for a long time. I wanted more joy, and as I have gone on in this journey, more and more joy has started erupting out of my soul from the deepest recesses. I think it had been closed off because life had been hitting me in the face so hard, so now I engage with that joy and doing the things that fulfil me.

I have wanted to get back on stage and do a performance, and I'm currently in a performance. It's the first one, so I'm learning lines, and it feels good it's something fun for me. I just know as soon as I get on that stage, a part of me that was dormant will awaken again.

I have also been experiencing music in a new way, allowing it to soothe my soul, or help me build up my energy to do a workout. Whatever kind of mood I need to be in music can help. Before music was just music but there are many pieces which can bring us healing, or the emotional release that we need in a moment.

I love listening to running water, which is weird, but Spotify has a great selection of running water sounds, so I am using music and sound to bring extra healing to my body and discovering a piece of myself that I shut down long ago because I had to do adulting and I believed I couldn't have fun anymore. This book is part of the fun I now have in my life, helping others to get breakthrough in their lives, by using my life and particularly my healing journey to teach them.

It's exciting to see what the future holds for you. My 80 year old self is going to look back at my 35-year-old self and say, "thank you for sorting your s**t out"

CHAPTER 8- OVERCOMING THE I AM NOT ENOUGH TRAP

Now let's talk about some of the hurdles that you may come up against when you embark on this journey that may feel like Mission Impossible, but where anything is possible. One of the biggest hurdles that I have had to overcome is fear of the unknown, fear of what is in my future. I am so scared of changing and not knowing what is going to happen from that change. I can see that this has come from being in my comfort zone for a longtime. It's our brains main task to keep us safe and away from danger, real or perceived. When it comes to making substantial changes, our brains can throw a little fit, an imposter syndrome can sneak in saying "who are you to do this?" "Why do you think you are good enough to help others?" That little voice that makes us doubt ourselves.

You and I both know that in a world that has so much to offer, we don't want to not be able to take opportunities that could give you a more fun and fulfilled life. What do you want for your kid/kids? Do you want them believing in themselves and feeling confident to take up opportunities? If the answer is yes it starts with you.

You have the power to start noticing what thoughts you are having more, and even why you may be having them and the key is to keep catching your thoughts.

Many of my clients have had to work through thoughts telling them they are not good enough. They feel like they are not enough for the world. They say they are trying and working, and they are making themselves so busy all the time that they can't be present for anything.

No one should feel like this, because you are enough in who you are right now, even before you change anything, and that is what we need to start believing.

You are good enough right now to learn how to take a break, and to give your body a rest, you deserve to stop for five minutes and have a peaceful, joy filled life.

You can become your very own cheerleader, and this has been the best gift I have given myself; I can celebrate my own wins when they happen. When others spot them and congratulate me as well it's like a double celebration in my brain.

I didn't believe I was enough being in our farming family. I believed that in order to fit in, in order to be good enough, I had to work really hard long hours and earn money normally in my second job off the farm. I believed it was how strong I was physically that was the key. When actually it's my brains not my brawn that's getting us further in life. I had this thought process because in the farming industry, if you're in it you will know there is constantly a financial element tied in, we never seemed to earn enough money for the hours we did. Many farmers have encouraged their children not to come back into farming, to go and find something else to do, another profession that is going to earn them some money and not have them working 12-14 hours a day 7 days a week sometimes.

Imagine what happened to my brain when I had Hayley and I thought, "it will be fine, I will be on maternity leave and then I'll go back to work". But I couldn't go back to any kind of physical work as I had before because of my injuries, and I had no extra money coming in that was my own. Thankfully I do have an amazing husband supporting us. He may read this one day! But it wasn't the same, all of a sudden "I wasn't good enough" because my DO was tied into my WHO which is an unhealthy view point.

It was about that time, Hayley was six or seven months old that I joined Tropic, and I started bringing in an income again. I used Tropic to basically make me feel like I was busy. I was earning money, and that money subsequently went towards me, and my treatments to help my physical health which I am grateful for because private treatments aren't cheap. But all my brain had done was work out another way that I could be busy and earn money, never letting me address the real problem, which was a very overactive, unproductive mind, creating exhaustion.

After a few years, I remember my mum telling me that I needed to pay more attention to Hayley. "She wants your attention, and you are constantly on the laptop". Straight away I shut the laptop, and Tropic started to go more on the back burner. At the time this was the right thing to happen, especially since our children grow up so quickly and we don't get this time again. But I remember feeling and being really annoyed! "why couldn't I do both?"

I loved selling Tropic and having a team, but it was just my brain covering over the fact that I hadn't dealt with the underlying problem, I was ignoring what my body was actually saying to me, and there was a whole heap that I needed to deal with.

I didn't want to go and see a counsellor because I thought there was nothing wrong with me, that I was fine. But I wasn't "fine" it could be a cover up for (f**ked up, idiotic, neurotic and emotional) according to a friend of mine and when he said it, I did laugh.

A big part of this journey is learning to allow the thoughts which keep you in the dark to come up into the light, so they no longer have any power over you. I imagine that whenever I write down a negative thought on a piece of paper, it brings it into the light and it shines so brightly, that I am able to deal with it quickly. The logical part of my brain looks at the thought and tells me "It is not true". My logical brain says, "how can you even believe that?". Not feeling loved, or speaking bad things about ourselves is something every woman I know seems to do, it's become such a habit we don't even know when we do it.

We all want to feel loved, and many of us have different ways of showing love. There are five basic ways that helps us to feel loved, to be able to give and receive love as well, these are the love languages.
Words of Affirmation, Acts of Service, Receiving gifts, Quality time, Physical touch.

If our needs have not been met emotionally as a child for whatever reason, this can roll into our teens, and then into our adult life. It is sad how it feels like for a few generations we have been on the wrong path with this, and we are now reaping the consequences of children being really unhappy and expressing that in very upsetting ways to us as parents.

I grew up in a family who loved me, took care of me and provided for me and they are still always there for me. However, our family was not great at connecting emotionally, we were not what you would call a "Huggy family". We loved each other and we would do anything for each other. If one of us was in trouble, another one will come and rescue us, and it was always like that. But there was an emotional level missing, which came through mental and emotional health trauma that my gran had been through and had affected my dad.

When I was doing this work in the very beginning with Hayley, I remember that when she was 18 months old, she started doing what 18-month-old babies should be doing. She was testing boundaries, she was trying my patience, she was making me angry, and I was losing it. I was getting so angry; she would pull my hair, and I would be screaming at her.

I think this went on until she was three years old. Then one day (it was a defining day), I picked up one of her dolls push chairs, and I smashed that push chair against a wall. I realised right then and there that I had got to do something about my anger. Anger is a powerful tool when used appropriately.

We need anger if our child has been wronged in some way, and if we need to fight for things we believe in, we need that anger to erupt. However, if our child is doing something that we deem to be wrong based on our past experiences, and we don't have the emotional intelligence to handle it and it is causing anger in us, it can cause a great divide within our child and our relationship with them.

This is what I was doing with Hayley, I was not allowing her to make mistakes, or to have a melt down because she was 3, without me acting like a 3 year old as well. If you find yourself getting angry a lot and then feeling guilt and shame afterwards this can be a sign that something is not right within your subconscious thoughts. That there is so much fear happening in your mind the resulting emotion is anger. That anger comes out on those we love the most because they are there and they just learn to take it.

We now know though that when we get to teenagers, we end up choosing to do the one thing that all parents are afraid of and that's rebel, because our connection is not secure. We shut down, we hide away from our parents in any way we can, and if we aren't careful we get ourselves into situations which are dangerous.

Why do we do this? Because if our emotions weren't being met calmly and in a rational way when we were toddlers and children and we were being shouted at or knew not to get upset because we didn't want to upset our parents, we end up not feeling loved. Ouch!

Showing love to our children, and ultimately to ourselves in the messy times of life is the best way of receiving and giving love and helps form strong attachments and relationships in the family. Where we feel like it's safe to talk, or have a meltdown sometimes is when the best communication and relationships can happen.

In fact in our house if I have a meltdown as I am working things through I am still human even after all, I know the best way I can model a healthy way to Hayley is by saying sorry quickly and explaining that mums can get upset and angry as well, and it's not because of her.

I have also a new built in thought process that allows me to feel when I am about to get to boiling point, and say to whoever is pushing the buttons, "I am getting this close to blowing my top (showing them with my fingers how short the fuse is) and often this is enough for the child to think "ok we don't want to go there" and do whatever it is I am asking them to do.

This chapter may have been a hard pill to swallow, these subjects can be gnarly and make us feel uncomfortable they can even set off a spiral of negative thoughts about how bad you are as a parent, or person etc....

This is a normal response to something when we are bringing the darkness into the light. The deepest thoughts we can harbour particularly about our parenting being read in black and white, is the next level of healing. Its allowing yourself to feel the feelings that have come up and decide right now that it stops with you. That these behaviours stop with you, and the work you are doing will bring blessings not only to your children's generation but your grandchildren and great grandchildren as well.

CHAPTER 9- BREAKING FREE FROM PERFECTIONISM

Perfectionism is another mindset which can cause us great anxiety and sometimes anger. Perfectionism has been an issue on my journey time and time again. Even writing this book, perfectionism pops up because it will say, "who are you to write a book? Why are you writing it? That's not right, you haven't said that right? That punctuation is not right" "You have repeated yourself a zillion times". Perfectionism for us is huge, and this can be because we have not been allowed to make mistakes and feel like it was ok afterwards.

Often situations happen and it all blows over but there are a few words not said, and these are often the most important, it's the ones that remind us its ok when we make mistakes. Often though as parents we don't have the time or even notice that we haven't reassured our kids, after a mistake. We are quick to point the mistake out, but it's not so easy to guide a child through the emotions of that and give them the words they need to hear, especially if we are triggered and in the heat of the moment angry.

Many of us have been shouted at, sent to our rooms, or punished in some way for making even a small mistake. But the thing is, all human beings need to make mistakes, this is how we learn. It's sad that we don't seem to be able to deal with mistakes that have been made in a rational and calm way We teach our children as toddlers to walk. They fall over, they get back up, they fall over, they get back up.

Isn't the falling over a mistake? We don't berate them for the mistake. But once they get to two, three, four years old, all of a sudden, it's not cute anymore.

We are fighting them every step of the way and we are stopping them from truly experiencing who they are. I had so many regrets about situations where I did that with Hayley, where she needed me to be stable, she needed me to show up, and I was not able to do that.

My own issues with perfectionism getting in the way and creating fear and anger. I didn't want to be someone who lived in regret, I know that the past is done, and I need to move on into the future. And the same is open to anyone who is willing to put the effort in and make the changes, for the sake of themselves and their kids.

This work I know will save such heartbreak for me when Hayley is a teen because we are connected so much better now, than we were. We can communicate our problems without one or the other of us getting angry. As for perfectionism I have learnt that it does nothing but cause more stress and strife, that each one of us have things we are good at we just need the confidence and often the encouragement of others to do something different.

If it's wrong, then you can start again or adjust and give it another go. I reckon that's what will happen with me and this book. The main aim though is it gets out into the world to start helping others know they can make life changing changes for their families.

I know that Hayley is now better equipped to deal with making a mistake than I was at her age, sadly the school system did that to me. She knows that if she makes mistakes, she can come to me and tell me about it. Most of the time I am completely chilled. If there is a situation, even in public, where she has had a meltdown for whatever reason, even at nine years old, she knows that 99 percent of the time, I will stay calm enough to get us through the situation. That wasn't happening when she was little, but it is never too late to change.

I can manage my own temper now, I can prevent my brain going into thought processes around being judged by others, which is often what mothers have whizzing around their minds when their kids are acting up in public. These feelings of being judged can also bring up angry feelings in a situation when you are trying to calmly handle things.

If we get angry then that's when our children can start to lose respect for us, they become scared of us, and they will start to not trust, or even listen to us because why should they? this is exactly what happened with Hayley and I.

Respect is mutual and needs to go both ways, we gain respect from our kids by helping them calmly through their problems no matter how little they are. In fact, if you can help your toddler with their big problems at the time, then your teenager will trust you with their big problems at the time which tend to be a little bit more to handle as they navigate through puberty and those challenges.

Hayley was not trusting me, and we still now must continue to build up that trust, we are in a position now where I know that she needs more structure in her learning.

I want her to be able to read and write effectively, things that have been a struggle since we took her out of school because it reminds her too much of school, and because she can't do it perfectly her perfectionism issues kick in.

She still isn't trusting me enough to see I am putting her into this situation for her own good, for her future and it can get a bit heated sometimes especially as she is a bright cookie and deep down, I know she just wants to be like "normal" kids and do these things, but we are working on it.

If you find yourself wondering as you read this through about your emotional health and how to identify your feelings the best sources, I have found are the Usbourne Book of Emotions. It has all the basics: happiness, calmness, anger, frustration, worry, anxiety. There is literally a page of children's faces expressing different emotions, and I picked it up one day and I thought, "have I ever learnt these things?".
I have another book called The Book of emotions by Tiffany Watt Smith, there are over 154 different emotions in it, it is amazing how humans are so beautifully complex and its even better that we now have more knowledge and information at our fingertips to learn about ourselves.

We as human beings need to reconnect with our emotions. Anger is there for a reason, yet when used in the wrong way, can cause the most harm. I have now learnt that saying sorry is a really good way of teaching your child how to say sorry when they have gotten angry. But it is also a really good way to rebuild trust. It shows your child that you are not perfect either, and I think this has been one of the main things that I have been able to model to Hayley.

The fact that I'm not perfect, you're not perfect, and we are living in this imperfect world together. We are just being the best we can be in that moment and working towards a different version of ourselves and that is okay.

If Mum is having a down day, then mum's having a down day, I can be having a really big meltdown, and Hayley is now so in tune with my emotions that she can come alongside me give me a hug and kiss, and tell me she loves me. Once she told me she was proud of me. This journey isn't easy, this journey has had me crying in the bathroom in the middle of the night at times, because I felt like screaming "what is wrong with me? Why do I think like this? Why do I feel like this?"

I have started to see clearer, and I have come into the light and realised that I don't need to be thinking this. I don't need to feel like this, there is a different way to think, feel and be.

I can just be myself, bring out all my weirdness if I want to, my excitement, my overflow of joy, that always used to be there as a child, my quick wits, my ability to make somebody laugh. This version of me should not get shut down because life happened and I became an adult, and it shouldn't happen in you either.

CHAPTER 10-COACHING VERSUS COUNSELLING

The difference between the coaching work I do, and counselling is vast. There may be a place for counselling on journeys like this, but it does not necessarily help create a future version of yourself.

With counselling you often have to go back into the past, and sometimes you can end up staying there, which isn't healthy and can sometimes cause more mental harm than good. If you're replaying traumatic things in your mind and you don't know how to fully release them. With coaching it's about creating a future vision or version of yourself that you may have never seen before.

A 2.0 version of you, where you get to decide in every area of your life how you are being, acting, what you are doing. From managing your time like a true boss, to eating a diet specifically for your body the power of being coached by a Neurocoach is limitless. Which is why I love doing it.

Through the steps of becoming the 2.0 version or I think I am probably on 4.0 by now, I have had to learn to release burdens or emotions that I have held onto for a variety of reasons.

Doing this with the focus of the future rather than the past has made sure I have done things slowly, it has been a bit like unpeeling an onion one layer at a time. My experience when I have been in a counselling situation has been that if you peel off too many layers at once it can cause huge mental health problems for a time.

I learnt this with my granny when I was unbeknown to me counselling her, and I didn't know that it's important to stop people before they get too deep into their past situations. In the end with my dear granny, I was able to coach her to see things differently, and in a positive and more exciting way for her after suffering from a life time of pain, she just didn't need or want to keep reliving it.

I am someone who feels a lot of other people's pain, their grief, their anguish and I of course feel deeply when tragic situations happen in my life, particularly when my grandad died suddenly. It took me nearly 8 years to let go of the grief, to release the muscle memory of that day so that it no longer has a hold on me. If I had gone to a counsellor soon after it had happened, I wouldn't have struggled for so long.

The fear of dying and death comes stark into reality when something like that happens, and the emotions of that time if not released can literally drive every decision you make from that point forward. You get stuck in the fear.

I have learned that I can let go, I can let go of what happened in the past, and I can focus more on the present and making decisions that ensure my future is bright, that Hayley's future is bright, and that we are doing things we love in a world that seems like it's set up to stop us and makes us afraid of everything.

When I first heard the saying "Failure is the seed to success", I thought it was a bizarre saying. But now as I look back, I can see that where I have failed, I am now the most successful. My past mistakes have now become the base I can create a new life on.

When I let go of Tropic for a few years, I felt I had completely failed. But letting go of that part of my life at that time opened a new part of being a mum to Hayley. Being present, helping her to be confident, more resilient, and build skills within her that could only come from me, because she needed me. I had to coach myself along the way!

Hayley once said to me "Can you back off a bit, it's a bit too much" Being an only child for her is hard because it's all about her. To me, her saying that was a defining moment, because it meant, "OK, my work being present in her life is being shown to her. I can let go a bit, I can continue to help her on her journey, but I don't need to be that person anymore. I can move forward and do the exciting things that I want to do, like writing this book and helping other women get the same breakthroughs that I have had with Hayley and in my life.

My health is another area that I have worked incredibly hard on changing how I think, it is still an ongoing process. Sometimes I see quick results when rewiring my thoughts, but other times I will have thoughts that block me from getting the results I want. In those times, I will speak to my coach to help clear that thought away. It can sometimes take minutes, hours or a few days for me to unstick the thought, but I will get there in the end, the more you do this work the easier it becomes.

My issues and thoughts around my weight have not yet produced the results I want. I want to be able to move around easier and wear smaller clothes. According to the doctor, I'm healthy.

I don't have diabetes or high cholesterol and there is nothing wrong with my liver. I was hoping that throughout my journey, I would have lost the excess energy my body is currently storing as fat, but the complete opposite happened. I have gained weight, I know there is a bigger reason, and a bigger story behind it, but I'm still working through it. I have given myself five years to work on my health, rather than 5 minutes and that feels good to even make that kind of decision. Making small steps towards a healthier future, rather than making big steps and it back firing on us which can often be the case with a weight loss journey.

We think that things must happen overnight, we need it instantly, we have got to hit that goal now. I have learned that I can set a goal but sometimes I don't see the results for six to twelve months, there are some goals I made 5 years ago, and I know I am making the steps towards hitting them one day. Sometimes it's not until I look back I realise I had reached my goal! I believe that we sometimes have to complete the hard steps first, in order to enable us to be strong and keep moving forward.

I do not want to allow myself to get burnt out again, unless its for good reason. I may love the instant results you can get, but the extreme process to get to that point right now would not be healthy for me. Those size 12 jeans can wait a bit longer!

CHAPTER 11-RESTORING YOUR ENERGY AND IDENTITY

This isn't a journey for the faint hearted. This is a journey for somebody who is dedicated to becoming the best they can be, the best mum they can be. Someone who wants to take care of themselves, by not allowing themselves to get exhausted or burned out, not allowing their brains, and their thoughts to run away with them. You have to be willing to capture your thoughts no matter how ugly they are.

Ten years ago I did not think I would be living the life I am today. I am grateful for every little thing that has happened along the way. I am grateful for all the challenges and hardship, because I know it will enable me to help more people in the future. When Hayley is driving and able to get herself around and says, "I don't need you anymore", I know I have something exciting to step into because I had created it in a vision 10 years previous.

That something is what I will have built over the years, nurturing her and taking care of her. As mums we are creating adults and we want them to be able to think rationally, keep calm and create healthy thriving families of their own, we know that they are going to leave us one day, and they are going to have their own life, and that is OK it's how it's supposed to be.

We have sown the seeds of life into them, we have given them good roots, but eventually it's time to let them bloom on their own. If there's a hurdle that you're going to hit on this journey, then I have probably hit it before you. If there is something that you are going to get stuck on, I can help you get unstuck, I can help you see the way around the problem, I can help you find another way or do what you need to do in that moment.

What is it, what is the secret key that helps us to live the life that we want to live? What is it that helps us to manage our time, have more energy and be present with our children and families that we can truly start to enjoy our lives? The secret truly is that you hold the answers. Deep inside of you, you know in your heart of hearts what you want your life to look like and you know what you want to be doing. However, we live in a world that seems and feels like it is set up against us at times. But we have the power inside of us to change things, for generations to come.

When we feel that whatever way we turn, we are not working hard enough, we are not good enough, we don't earn enough money. We all struggle with guilt to some degree, and this means that it can become hard for us to see our lives being any different than what they currently are.

We all want to have a peaceful and organised life that is busy, but in a fun easy way. To have a life that gives us energy and life, not one that drains our energy and makes us so exhausted that our bodies basically disown us and eventually make us sick, physically, emotionally or mentally.

Many people, particularly women in the world, struggle with time management, we can't sit down for a five-minute cup of tea without having that nagging feeling in our head, "I should be doing something". Then thinking of the list, the never-ending list that mums seem to have, it means that we never truly get rest. Even when we're on holiday, many of us can struggle because there's other things we need to take care of. Our brain is so busy, running wild with us.

One day I was sat in my room, and I knew that I was onto something when I had complete quiet in my brain. It was the weirdest feeling, because I honestly do not remember when the last time that had happened. I sat there for just a few moments before my brain started pinging again. Ping in a thought, ping in a song, and from that moment on, I knew that it was possible to quieten my mind enough to be able to think properly, not just think from a place of fear all the time.

Many of us are scared, and we wonder why we're so scared. Or we don't wonder why we are scared, because we haven't even noticed that most of the daily actions and words we speak are from a place of fear. This means that we make choices that are not going to be good for us in the future. I can trace back to where I have made decisions, and taken action on situations that have caused me harm. They have tired me out, they have taken a lot of my health away from me, and that meant when it came to being a mum I really struggled.

I was so afraid of messing it up, I was so afraid that I had to be good enough, I had to do do do! I remember that during the time I couldn't walk properly, I was grateful for that time because it meant I could spend time with my baby. Those first twelve months it was literally just her and I, little did I know then that we would end up back there again when we started home educating. For most of the time we are together and that is a great blessing to me.

I have messed up so many times, but then I have known exactly how to deal with the mess and it often turns our better than before, just imagine a world for our kids where this is the case. Can you see it? Feel it? Do you want it?

CHAPTER 12- LEARNING TO BE BETTER ROLE MODELS FOR OUR KIDS

One of the other challenges that mum's have is, if we have never had a role model, how do we know how to do certain things? How do we get this life? There are lots of resources out there, books, films, courses, groups, many things out there to try and help you get the life you want. However, if they aren't the steps that you need for your life right now, they can make things a whole lot worse for you. You can end up in a place where the wheels are spinning and your feeling overwhelmed, not knowing where is best to start, or what to do next.

By looking at what you want your life to be like, and creating a vision for what you want it to look like in the future, you can make better decisions so that you can become the role model for your family. I know that I am a great role model for Hayley and the other children who I am blessed to have in my life, I am even a pretty good role model now to adults in my life as well.

This has always been one of the most important things to me. How do I want to show up for Hayley? How do I want to show up for the rest of my family? I want to make better decisions now, so that my family's future is better.

But thinking about it used to make me feel so overwhelmed that I didn't know where to start. As I said before, being overwhelmed is another way our brain can block us and stop us making changes to our lives.

You may read this book and feel so overwhelmed by thoughts saying, "I can't do any of this!" This is because your brain is filled with "I can't and I won't and I don't", and it can stop you in your tracks and you never get out of the rut. Your heart might be saying "but I really want a different way of living" but your brain is saying "no, sorry it's not safe". There is so much more to life than having a brain that is over stimulated, and over worked, which makes the rest of your body feel completely exhausted.

It may sound like what I am offering and what I'm saying to you is impossible. But we now know how the brain works, and just like other things that we didn't know about in the past, knowledge on how things work increases. Once upon a time there was only horses and carts on the roads, but somebody somewhere had the idea to create a car because they believed they could create something better.

It's the same for families. If you want to create something, you must first believe that you can create it, and then be able to make it happen through your decisions and actions. Time management is important as we all need to be able to manage our time well, so that we have more energy. Then we can see what we want to do. Managing our time better allows us to see quickly the positive results of rewiring our thoughts and helps us gain some much-needed extra energy which isn't being burnt by the brain anymore.

Once we are unstuck from our own thoughts, we can help other people unstick theirs. Once we are running the race we can reach back and see if we can help anybody else, that is essentially what I am doing, I am saying, "come on! We can run the race together!" That is what human beings are for, we are here to help each other, work with each other and be with each other.

The sooner we work out that it is the state of our mental and emotional health which is telling us we have to do everything by ourselves when we don't, the sooner the world around us can get to a place of pure bliss and be enjoyable again. We need community and we need connection with others.

Community and Connection

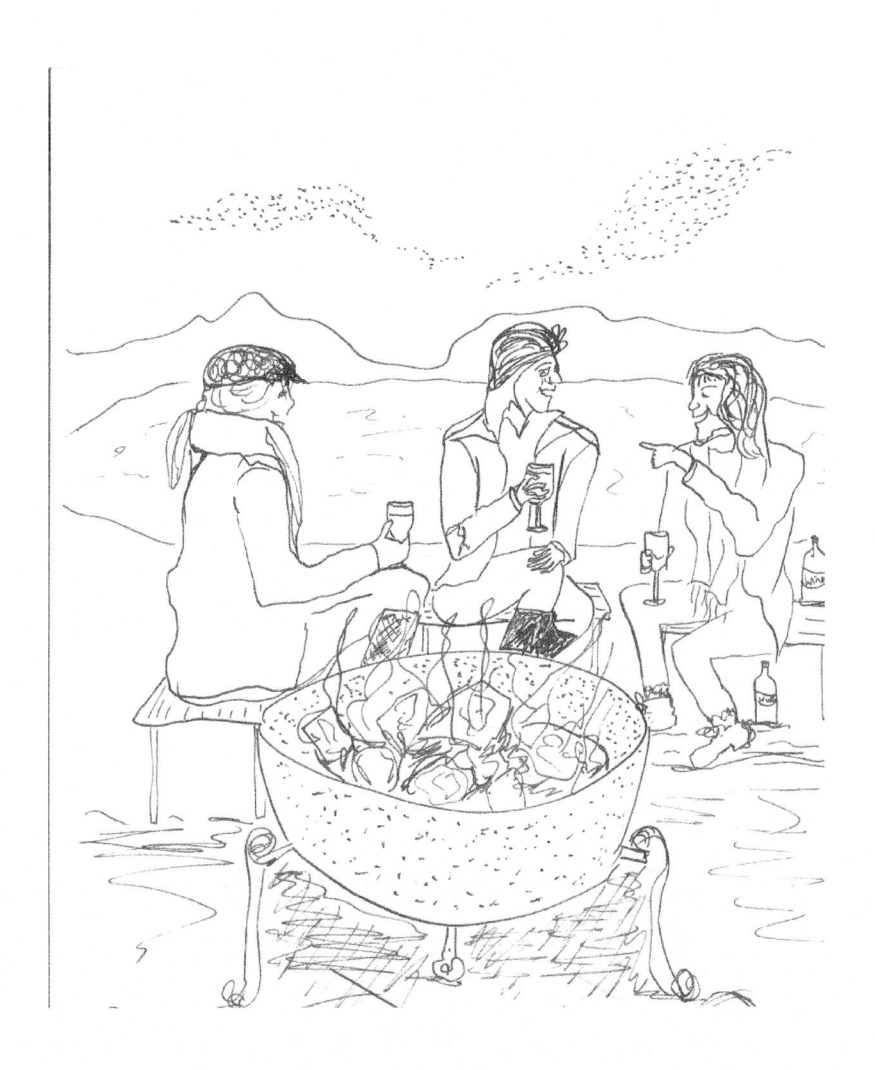

CHAPTER 13- WHEN YOU TRY EVERYTHING AND NOTHING STICKS

If you're anything like me, you will have tried many different things to have a different lifestyle. You have tried self-help books, health plans, you've tried to have better time management. You want to have the skills to be able to keep a better diary, or if you are thinking you may have ADHD which is something I identified in myself. You may think "I will never be able to do this, I will never be able to change".

However, what is exciting is our brains have so much potential. My brain works so fast with so called ADHD, there is nothing deficient about me, I have been able to imagine the life I want to have, and I am seeing what I can achieve when my brain is working at speed on what I WANT it to. Somewhere along the lines brains just get a bit disorganised, but we can change that now and its backed by science making it easier and more accessible for the likes of you and I, who don't have a PhD in Neuroscience.

Time management skills, looking after myself first, my health, eating, drinking, moving and sleeping well, all the things which enable me to have a healthy and balanced life.

To be able to be present and not have our brains over thinking, especially whilst we are with people. How amazing is it going to be when you achieve these things and have a brain that is working for you rather than against you, because this already makes a huge difference in my life.

Before I started this work, I thought I had tried everything. I did course after course, I had read books and articles about all sorts of things to do with health and time management, how to be a good mum, how to be more present and engaging. I had read and watched lots of videos, yet nothing seemed to work out for me, I was still exhausted and getting nowhere. Nothing seemed to stick.

When I joined Dr Shannon Irvine with her Neuro-coaching programme though, I realised it was because I was not utilising the most powerful asset I have, and that is my very own brain. My brain was full of thoughts that didn't need to be in there, as I have shared with you, and I would guess that your brain has the same problem, it needs a little tidy up. Mine was like a giant bomb had gone off.

Remember this exercise, if you haven't done it already. Take a pen and paper and set an alarm for 20 minutes, and write down every thought that you have in those 20 minutes. Then I want you to look at what you wrote. What does it say about what is going on in your mind. When I did this myself, I realised why I was so tired. I had to burn that piece paper because I never wanted anyone to see it.

When we are learning to capture our thoughts, we learn to visualise what we are thinking. We can bring our sub conscious thoughts up into our conscious. Once our thoughts are captured, only then can we design the life we want to have and reach our goals. There will be some big thought processes in your brain that if you manage to catch them and see what they are, you are going to be able to change your whole life for good. This is not just a quick fix, but lasting change.

I'm not saying that anybody else's solution is wrong, but I have learned that if it's not the right solution at that time, you could be setting yourself up to fail. Dieting is a big one for this, *(more to come on that in the next book.)* This is called self-sabotage where your own brain makes decisions and actions which make you fail, and then you end up with a flurry of negative self-talk which does nothing for your health or your stress levels.

I have even witnessed that a person's brain can be so used to running on energy by saying horrible things about themselves that they will create situations so they can say more horrible things about themselves. It sounds weird doesn't it, but this is what happens when our minds and our throughs have become undisciplined in certain areas of our lives.

This is why it helps to have a coach walking you through the process and having a coach who has been through the same process, I am practicing what I preach here, and I know I can help you get quicker results, to have more time more energy and enjoy life.

To learn all the steps of rewiring your brain, working with someone trained to show you all the steps to do it is a powerful tool. Another tool needed is the desire to do it. The desire to go on the journey, why would you want to change your life? What areas do you just wish things were different in?

Most of what I have done has been through pen and paper, but there are also big decisions in my life that I have had to work through with a coach, purely because they see the things that I do not, they see what is blocking me.

This is done by listening to the words that are coming out of my mouth and repeating them back to me. You will never believe how many things people say, and when you repeat them back to them, they can't believe they have said it, or they can't believe that they have that belief even.

I do this with my dad all the time, the poor chap, he doesn't ask me to coach him, but he gets it anyway he doesn't realise how much I am helping him change his life just yet, but one day he will.

In essence, nothing is impossible anymore with the knowledge we have about our fascinating brains, it should be the key focus in our parenting, that we are helping a little brain develop into an adult brain, and they all need a different approach, which miraculously we as their mums can know how to handle. We were designed that way.

When our messy unorganised brains get in the way though it can leave us feeling stressed, burnt out and taking it out on the very people we don't want to be taking our crap out on.

CHAPTER 14- WHAT IS YOUR WHY?

The key to making sure what I am sharing with you can work for your life, and doesn't turn out to be another block, is motivation and your why. Why you are doing this? Why do you want to change your situation and who do you want to change it for?

One of the main parts of this process I have found is to realise what my life is now. For me, my life since she was born has been about my daughter Hayley, and helping her become a happier and healthier child. As soon as she was born, I held her in my arms, and I knew that I didn't want her to feel anything like I had ever felt, so she became the clean page I needed to rebuild myself. Every hard decision I have had to make, every process I have been through, every tear I cried was for her, and for myself. I want to be a good role model, and I want to feel free in myself.

Why is it so important for you to go on this journey? It's hard when we are going through periods where our brain is starting to create new neural pathways, it can feel daunting. You may be doing this for your family. I have seen my mum work hard, and always putting others before herself, which has led to her health problems now, which we are working on changing.

I have health problems myself, and I didn't want to be like it, I didn't want to stay stuck thinking this was it. Our work hard and not take care of ourselves ethic caused both my mum and I to not have good health. I was 24 when it happened my mum was 57. It doesn't have to be that way we don't have to stay stuck being unhealthy and stressed in pain and on medication if we don't want to.

What would your 80-year-old self-thank you for, what is within your power to change now particularly in your health so you don't become a burden to your kids or family in the future? This is my driving force, because I have mobility issues, the longer I leave it the worse it would get so I am dealing with it now, and I know exactly what steps I need to take every day! Guess why? Because I have trained my brain by creating a vision of the fully healthy me. I have created something in my mind that's in the future, and I have brought it into the present so my daily actions and decisions work towards the vision of a fully healthy me.

I want you to have a think about you, "why?" Why do you want to change your life? Why do you want to stop being burned out? Why do you want more energy? It is more than possible for you to do what you want to help the people in your life. The next bit is working out how to do it in the best and quickest way possible.

The Seven Why's Exercise

Grab a piece of paper, I want you to write down the very first thing you think of when I say:

Why do you want to Reclaim your time, boost your energy and rediscover a new you in the process?

Then I want you to ask yourself why to this answer and write that down.
Then I want you to ask yourself why to this question and write down the answer
Then I want you to ask yourself why to this question and write down the answer
Then I want you to ask yourself why to this question and write down the answer
Then I want you to ask yourself why to this question and write down the answer
Then I want you to ask yourself why to this question and write down the answer

It may get a little tricky around the 4th/5th why but sit with it and wait for your brain to give you an answer. When you get to the end of this process, this is your real why. This is the why that connects with your heart not just your head and it's the one you need to write down and stick somewhere. This is going to help you to keep going.

CHAPTER 15- YOUR VISION FOR THE 2.0 VERSION OF YOU

This is it, this chapter is about how you are going to be able to live a life that you are not burnt out from, how you can manage your time better as well as do all the wonderful things that satisfy you.

The first part, as I mentioned in the previous chapter, is to discover your why. Why are you doing this? It could be someone you want to make changes for, or something specific in your life, like your health. You need to have a good think about your "why"? Because this is going to give you the motivation and ability to keep going through this process.

The next thing you need to do is create your vision. Do you want more time? Do you want to feel healthier? Do you want to feel more relaxed? Imagine what it looks like, feels like and smells like to be the 2.0 version of you. Make sure you add as much detail as you can, make it as full and big as you can. It is exciting as it is your creation and vision. Add in any hopes and dreams you may have had over your lifetime that you have not yet seen happen.

I have put 50 "Vision Spark" examples at the back of the book. Your vision needs to be written in present tense like it already happened. Use "I am statements". When you have done this, grab your phone and record what you have written. You can then use an app called TLC to help you put your vision prime on repeat and start listening to it in the mornings and evenings and any other time of the day you think about it. The sooner you get to 67 listens the sooner your brain will create its new neural networks and you start seeing results.

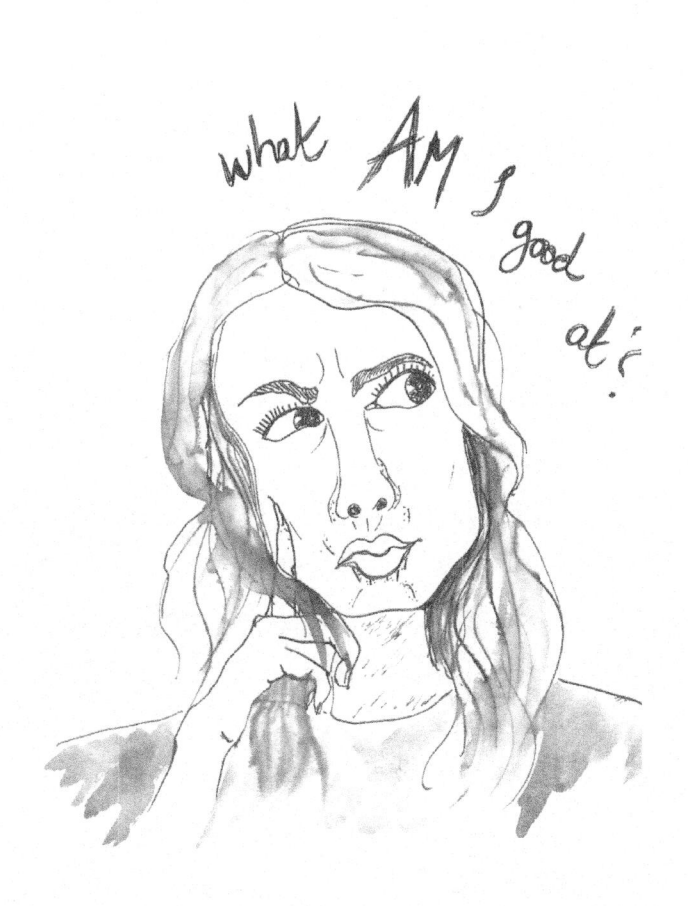

The next step is noticing your thoughts and what your brain is saying about this vision that you have created? When you read through the 2.0 version of your vision what does your brain say? Remember you don't believe these things yet. It takes a minimum of 67 listens of this vision before your brain can make it a new belief system for you.

In the meantime, there will be brain blocks! I have added a big list of some of these at the back of the book, but the chances are you may be having way more than the ones I have mentioned.

To capture them, use a pen and paper, I have one with me all the time, or I use notes on my phone. Using a phone doesn't quite have the same effect as there is connection between your sub conscious and writing things that you don't tap into when typing. Just bare this in mind if you want to get down into the deep nitty gritty of your sub conscious and bring about these lasting changes.

I also learned how to pay attention to what my body is doing. The body is constantly giving you feedback that you can use to help you with your transformation. For example, if I'm a bit worried about something, I will start breathing heavily, I will start getting warmer and sweating, I may feel a heavy lump in my chest, or in my stomach.

These are key markers to what emotions are going on behind your thoughts. It is your emotions that can stop you go forward or help you go forward into a new version of you. It is important to start tuning into your body, maybe in a way you never have before.

When I sense a change in my body I will think "what just happened? what am I thinking about that has just caused me to be worried or often stressed". Then your brain will show you what you are thinking in that moment.

When you first start this, it might be slightly overwhelming because you'll have so many thoughts coming to the forefront, and your brain will be like, "oh, this, this, and this ", you may think "well that's not doing any harm", but those familiar thoughts are often the ones causing the most harm and using up the most energy. This is what is making you feel so exhausted.

Write all the thoughts down, They don't have to be in any kind of order, they don't have to make sense, you NEVER have to show them to anyone just write down exactly what you hear or visualise.

If what is coming out is too much and you never want to read them again burn them. I have had wonderful times with Hayley burning all the negative thoughts I have had in the past. It's been such a cathartic release, I first learnt about it in 2017 when I decided to write a letter to my grandad who died suddenly. It was the first steps to getting complete closure, from those intense emotions of grief and fear.

Capturing every single thought is one of the most powerful things that we can do on this journey.

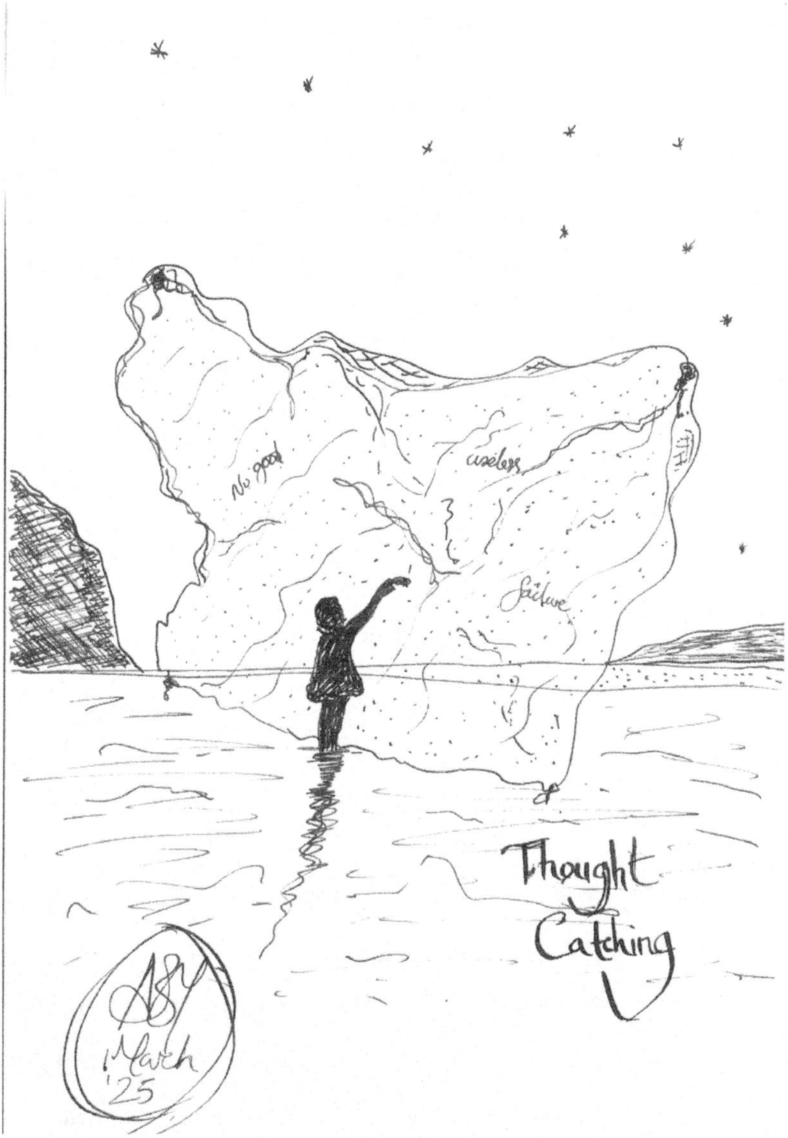
No good
useless
failure
Thought
Catching
1 March
'25

The next part is, what emotions are you feeling?

Do you know what emotions you are feeling? Do you realise you can change your emotions? You can go through one, two or three different emotions in just 15 minutes, depending on what your circumstances are at the time.

Do you feel shy?
Are you feeling jealous?
Are you angry?
Are you happy, calm, peaceful, sad, excited?
Are you anxious?
Are you feeling brave?

I have added a more extensive list to the back of the book, including where you feel them in your body.

Whatever the emotion is, we need to notice our feelings, and where we are feeling it. Are you feeling it in your head, your heart, your stomach, are you feeling it in your fingers? Tuning in and identifying it is what helps us to reconnect with ourselves and allows us to see what is going on in our bodies. We SHOULD have learnt to do this as kids, but these feelings have often been suppressed using plasters, Calpol or worse still do you want some sweets?

Our thoughts and emotions are intertwined, science says that when we have a thought, it creates an emotion. The one that many of us seem to relate to the most is anger sadly but that doesn't have to be the case.

Sometimes we get angry but have no idea why we are angry. It's because a situation can happen, someone walks into a room you don't like, someone sends you a message and you take it wrong, sometimes a smell could even trigger the thought to pop into our head unbeknown to us even and anger is felt. This is why identifying our emotions and learning about them is so important. It helps us take huge steps towards inner healing, and peace

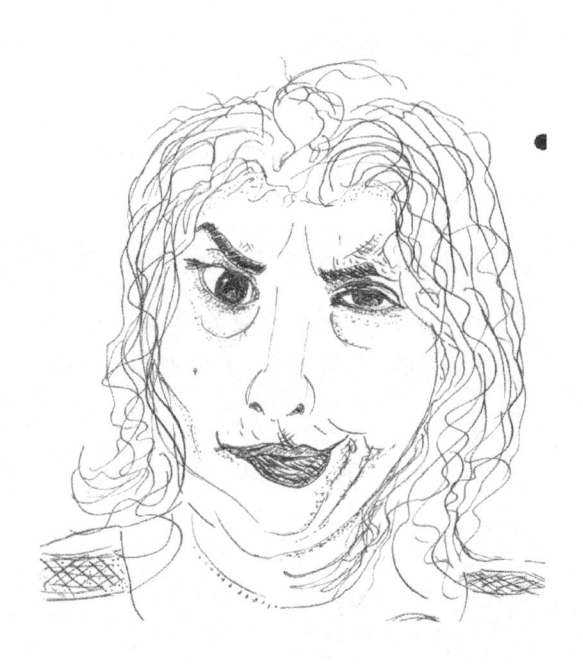

CHAPTER 16- BUILDING HEALTHY BOUNDARIES

Next up boundaries. Do you have any boundaries? Do you have emotional boundaries?

Many of us do not have emotional boundaries because we have not been shown what they are, or the people we have lived with don't have good ones to model to us. For me it was my inability to say no. I would say yes to everything and then feel overwhelmed.

There are other emotional boundaries, people can say and do things that you don't like. They could just barge into your room, or they could say something that triggers you and you don't know how to stop them doing it. Sayings like "she is a door mat" comes to mind or everyone else's happiness comes before yours"

What are your emotional boundaries?

What boundaries do you need to put in place to make sure you are keeping your energy safe, and not feeling triggered by negative situations all the time?

Creating boundaries is a great skill to teach our children.

I have taught Hayley not to allow people to speak to her in a certain way or touch her in a certain way, and that she can have a rest and sit on the sofa without feeling guilty. I am also teaching her that when someone says something horrible to her its often a sign of something going on in them like jealousy, it's not necessarily her fault.

I have shown her and allowed her to look after herself and rest. It's hard for me as I was used to always being busy, but I am changing myself now to be a good role model for Hayley and subsequently for other women in the generations to come. I don't want them to feel how I did about myself for 20 years.

This is such an important step on this journey. Being able to speak the words we need to create emotional boundaries. This can come through the beauty of brain priming, its where you show your brain what it is you want as simple as saying "I have good emotional boundaries and relationships with people in my family and my friends." And your wonderful brain will show you how to act and what to say to make sure the boundaries are being made and met.

We can choose our friends, but we can't choose our family. Sadly, they are often the ones who trigger us the most. It's important to know what to say, and how to say it to not cause anger and upset. It took me a long time to do this. Being able to say, "you've really hurt me by saying that", helps you to set an emotional boundary with your family and friends. It helps their brain to see that how they are behaving and what they are saying is hurting you.

CHAPTER 17- THE CHALLENGES NEW BRAIN WIRING CAN CREATE

When on this journey, your brain could become overwhelmed and feel it's not safe, these are what I call red flags. It is because your brain is so used to thinking and feeling a certain way, it isn't comfortable feeling anything different. Together we can work through the tough bits to get the results you want quickly, more time, more energy, and less money than what it cost me.

One of the things that I have struggled with is changing my eating habits but also changing what I eat. My brain for whatever reason has gotten comfortable with certain foods to get certain feedback from. It decides to do this when I introduce different meals and different flavours. I can often get the thought of this is poisonous don't eat anymore, with all the emotions that come with it. Recently I've been quite poorly and even the smell of cauliflower can trigger it's poison response.

I therefore have to tell my brain, "hang on, we can change our diet, we need to change our eating so that we can be healthier" This has been a slow process, but I am in control now of what I eat rather than just eating unconsciously and not noticing like before.

Another red flag could be that you feel angry or upset. You may feel like you can't do this anymore, like there is even more chaos than normal in your brain, or like there is cotton wool in there nothing at all. When I get to that point, and you don't know what else to do. That is when you know the breakthrough is coming in fact it's just around the corner. You have reached the messy, magical middle part of creating a new thought process.

This is often when I decide to message my coach, I'll say "my brain is telling me I can't do this, please help!" they will message back and ask me a question, or we will jump on a Zoom call. They will help me to see clearer and know what action to take next and to work through any big emotions which are coming up. Just taking a deep breath, and placing your hand on your chest can be the difference between overwhelm and calm in a matter of moments, it only takes 90 seconds of feeling all the "feels" remember to get them out of your body.

When I feel I cannot do this, that I am never going to do this or that it's too hard, I know that I am in a good place, because it means my brain is moving forward and is changing and adapting.

I also say "I don't know", a lot when I am in the middle of making a new thought process. I love it when I am coaching ladies and we get to an I don't know, because that's when I know we are close to a new breakthrough moment.

Trusting the Process is key.

These are the main steps I use to make sure that I am moving forward every day, creating the life I have designed not just one that is happening around me. I continue to home in on certain areas, being better at planning, sleeping better, eating healthier and managing both our farm business and my Tropic business in a productive way.

If I feel something is stopping me moving forward, I show my brain the changes I want to make through listening to my brain prime, I still make them regularly. The impossible becomes possible. If you believe it with all your heart, then you can create it. You don't have to see to believe right away, you must believe it to then see it! This is how you create an extraordinary life

CHAPTER 18- CHOOSE YOUR VILLAGE WISELY

Choosing who I spend my time with has been a big part of my journey. There are many people in our lives who speak negatively and bring us down, and they don't even know they are doing it. They may say things that aren't very funny, they may gossip or slander about other people in our lives, and you get the feeling they probably do the same about you when you aren't there. It can make life harder if you are surrounded by negativity, but you get to choose your boundaries now, remember you are an adult and can take back control of your energy and stop the energy vampires. I am fortunate that I have the right people with me at the right time, in fact part of this process is when we attract the very people we need when we need them.

I love positive encouraging people, but I need them to hold me accountable and don't let me get away with giving up and know that sometimes I need some tough love. This is especially true in my role as a Neuro-coach I will hold anyone who wants a transformation and is doing the steps accountable, to enable them to get unstuck. There is nothing worse than when someone thinks they are helping you by sympathising when you need them to kick your butt. My mum does this to me when I am having tough days.

Sometimes you may come across people who don't encourage you, instead they to do the exact opposite. They will say "this will never work, why are you bothering? what is the point of this?" It makes me angry just writing this knowing you may encounter these people, but ultimately, they are speaking to you from their own fears and faulty thinking, and it doesn't have to be that way. We get to choose how we think, feel and act, and if you want to discover a different way of living then you do that for you. And put your boundaries in.

For this to work, you need to find people who are going to encourage you and be there with you every step of the way, when you are crying, when you are screaming, when you feel meh and you just need a hug.

Next up Creating your village

Who is in your village? Maybe there are one or two people in your life that you need to step away from for the time being. Who are the people you need and want around you? These people will help you create the best life for your family. We live in a world that tells us, "mum's should be able to do everything all by ourselves", but it is not the truth. Humans need humans and different aged ones at that.

Children and families have always been in villages, not by themselves. I have a big family; we all live in one block with five kids and nine adults. We are a village, we always know that when something goes wrong, someone is going to be able to help us out.

My village is also bigger than my family, I have my church family, and I have my friends who are special to me and have impacted my life in one way or another. Many of those people have helped me stay safe when I was doing stupid things as a teenager. They are part of my village, and I feel fortunate to have them. I know that as I go on this journey, I am growing my village as well and new people will get added in and some will go, which is always sad but sometimes necessary.

Since becoming a coach, I have now got another new village! They are mainly in America, and they are amazing women who I owe a lot to for helping me get to where I am today.

Who is it you want in your village? How do you want your village to feel? How do you want it to look? Just considering the prospect of sharing your life with like-minded people is uplifting.

It doesn't need to be lots of people, it can be just a handful who will always have your back.

The next thing that you need is to have some self-compassion, to give yourself some grace, because you won't get it right the first time. It may take weeks, months, or even years of doing this work, but once you have got the framework which I have given you, and you know how to do the steps, you can use it for the rest of your life and create a life that you are proud of.

Self-compassion, again is something we haven't learnt, particularly as women. Everything is piled on top of us, we then put ourselves at the bottom of that pile and we don't take care of ourselves. We don't do things for ourselves, we don't manage our time well enough to be able to sit down and have a cup of tea and 5 minutes peace even. If you start having compassion for yourself, you are also becoming the best role model to your children, particularly girls. This is something we must be so aware of to make sure that our daughters and our sons know how to take care of themselves and be in tune enough with their bodies, to keep themselves healthy and happy and thriving.

Learn how to take a compliment! One of the very first steps I took towards self-compassion was changing how I reacted to compliments. I would often brush it off by saying something like, "what this old top? I bought it years ago", or I would ignore it completely if someone said I looked lovely.

Instead of doing this, I started saying "thank you". I started seeing that other people saw good things in me, that I wasn't seeing in myself. They thought I looked good, and they thought I was a good person. They could see that what I was doing was for a good reason. It was challenging to say thank you and acknowledge that other people saw the good in me.

When I started this journey, I was not very compassionate with myself. I had such a negative dialogue going on in my head. I was constantly berating myself, constantly telling myself that I was not good enough, or pretty enough. All the things that many of us have grown up thinking and believing.

When I started acknowledging compliments, I noticed a shift in how I felt about myself. This ultimately has helped me to show Hayley how to learn to love herself, from her hair to her heart and everything in between.

CHAPTER 19- FAILURE IS THE KEY TO SUCCESS

Being successful looks different to every one of us. The challenge we have is what successful means. When you have been through the formal schooling system particularly in the UK, you are taught that success is the end goal or the outcome, and you can often feel you must do it all perfectly.

When you took your exams, you were never encouraged to just enjoy the journey, to love and have fun in all the steps in between. This meant that we were often thinking about the future all the time and the end outcome, we were never present in the moment. This puts so much pressure on us, we can sometimes not cope or our perfectionism is so bad we just don't do anything in case we fail at it. So what if you do?

In my eyes, the end or the outcome for me is the day I go to heaven, none of us get out of here alive! which is hopefully a long way off, but before then I want to think I have lived the best life possible and enjoyed it, even the sad parts, because that's the joy of being human.

I didn't want the pressure of thinking I needed to do something and get somewhere all the time, I wanted to learn to enjoy the journey. Now that Hayley is eleven, I can see how those years have literally whipped on by. I wanted to be able to connect with her and enjoy the moments in her childhood. I have been able to enjoy this even more since we have been home educating. Hayley will be fully grown sooner than I think.

I have failed at things more times than I would like to admit, but I think it would be sadder if I hadn't given those things a go in the first place to see if I could do it. This process hasn't been linear at all. I have made some bad decisions especially when it comes to my health, I have made myself worse in some cases. And that's ok, it's not ideal but I trust that it can be fixed, it just may take a little bit of time.

Another area I have made some major mess ups in is business, writing this book, creating courses, email lists, marketing and funnels. All things I didn't have any skills to do a few years ago. I have tried and tried and tried again and I think I may finally be at a good point of its starting to work out. Perfectionism still tries to creep in. This book has been the worst for triggering it, its taken me months to get it together even with lots of help.

Setting new boundaries is going to be the same, a lot of trial and error. It can be quite hard to know what boundaries need to be put in place. Many of us need to choose to forgive the people that have hurt us. This is a really hard thing to do when we feel bitterness towards them, but it can cause us more harm than it causes them. An invisible force comes into play, and it isn't good for us.

There will always be those underlying feelings of anger and anxiety. I know I felt this with my dad. I am working on this and making progress. Our relationship now has become easier and more how I want it to be. We can chat with one another without falling out. We both now have new boundaries that we don't overstep, it's a two-way street. We have also learnt to say sorry to one another, which is a big thing.

Having boundaries regarding your time is also important. As a farmer's daughter, we had no boundaries at all with time. We would work all hours and be out at all times of the night when we really didn't need to be. We believed that this is what we had to do.

Nobody was checking up on us, so I don't know why we thought we had to do it! It was the same at weekends. We have had to put in strict times where we go and check all the animals of course, but there are periods within the year that all the animals are outside. So now we just nip round on those days to check them, and then we have the rest of the day off.

Time boundaries within families are important. I know that other people will have really bad time boundaries where you don't factor in anytime to rest at all. I always like to have hours in certain days where I can do nothing. If I want to go and have a little nap, or chill for a few hours, I can do it rather than making life so busy all the time. You can do this too, you're allowed to stop.

Sometimes Hayley and I like to have a film day. We will sit there all day and watch back-to-back films or watch a series. Having time boundaries is key to making sure that you don't get burnt out. The object of our lives is not to get burnt out as soon as possible, it is to have a healthy, happy, fulfilled life.

To do that, we must take back our time. We must notice what we are doing, recognise what we are spending our time on. It is as simple as tuning into our brains, our thoughts, and how we are perceiving the world

CHAPTER 20 - SLOWING DOWN TO SPEED UP

Slowing down to speed up. Now I have to say this is one of my favourite tips. You slow your brain down to ticking over speed, then you will find the right next steps to take. I do this at times in life when I feel like I am on a treadmill or a roller coaster.

If you feel you are getting nowhere, use this technique to stop you feeling overwhelmed. When our thoughts are racing, we don't make good decisions.

Once a friend said to me that we should only have one thought at a time, when she said it, I felt it was an impossible thing to do. But since then, I have realised that I am in control of what I think and feel. I have been able to change a lot of the negative thought patterns I had and finally reach a point where I have no thoughts at all. Its silence and peaceful in there, and that's when the real magic happens, and I have new ideas I never had before about parenting, business or farming, its cool!

I become more creative and can plan the next stages of what to do in my businesses normally, or what I need to do for my health. It's in the silence I have my biggest breakthroughs, how opposite to the world right now is this?

It was such a revelation to me when I first had brain silence. At the time my brain panicked and suddenly put a whole lot of thoughts in my head and music. It was then I realised that I was onto something, and I could have peace in my mind. I didn't need to be thinking all the time. Hayley even picks up on it, and she'll say, "mum you are over thinking, you don't need to think so much about that". When she says that, it helps me realise what I am doing.

"Why am I over thinking? "I'll ask myself. Asking myself questions has been one of the most profound things that I have discovered along the way, because when I start asking myself questions, my brain will often give me the answer. If we have a problem, we can ask ourselves "why do I have this problem?". Then often our brain will tell us. It is fascinating to me how this happens.

In a world where everything is about being busy and doing things as fast as possible, saying "I am slowing down to help myself speed up" sounds ridiculous.

There are times when I know I need to have slow seasons, I am writing this currently in the autumn which is a slower season for me. I have just come out of my fast season during the spring and summer. I have naturally chosen to do this so that in the spring I can hit the ground running, full of energy from being recharged. Fully rested from having taken care of myself.

CONCLUSION

So here we are. we have come to the end of our time together; I hope that you have enjoyed reading through this book. Just as a recap, I want to remind you that you are not alone, and you don't have to do things by yourself.

The key steps from this book

Take 10 minutes to write out all the thoughts you can catch in your mind

Create your own vision of your future, your 2.0 version with as much detail as you can. Record it on your phone and listen to it.

Do the seven whys exercise, to help give you the motivation to keep going

We all need a village around us, think about your village and the people who are going to encourage you and lead you in a powerful way.

Key things to remember

Your happiness is handmade, you get to choose what it is you want to be doing in your life, so that you feel happy and complete.

Your guiding light to life is deep within your own heart. Deep down in your heart you know what you want your life to look like. The challenge we have is that the world around us is so chaotic and is constantly bombarding us with things we need to be doing.

Your time is your own, therefore you should be choosing what it is you want to do with it, not someone else. You get to choose what you do with your time.

We all need to learn to slow down to help us become more productive and speed up. Slowing down our thought processes and our lives enough so that we can see the way we need to go.

Self-compassion is key, we can train our brain to be successful in whatever area of life we want to be successful. Whether that is self-care, parenting, our work life or our relationships with family and friends.

We can spend time on hobbies and the things we love to do, we are allowed. Adults are allowed to have fun.

I really hope and pray you have gotten something out of this book, I hope it helps you to move on to the next steps of your journey. Wherever you are right now, I hope that you have realised that you are the one in the driving seat of your life.

If you have used some of the steps I have mentioned and thought "Yes this is me!" I would love to hear from you! You can either email me or directly message me on social media, details at the back.

I am just a mum who has discovered a different way of living, and I want to share that with you. I know how difficult it is when you desperately want to do everything for everyone, yet you find yourself feeling exhausted.

Appendix 1- Vision Sparks

Time & Energy Freedom

1. I am waking up refreshed and ready for the day.
2. I am enjoying quiet time for myself before the kids wake.
3. I am winding down peacefully each evening.
4. I am clear on my daily priorities without overwhelm.
5. I am protecting guilt-free time just for me.
6. I am moving through my days without rushing.
7. I am ending the day with energy to read, journal, or connect.
8. I am resting and recharging at weekends.
9. I am saying "no" with confidence and kindness.
10. I am enjoying family life without the constant pressure.

Health & Body Reset

11. I am cooking simple, nourishing meals with ease.
12. I am feeling confident and vibrant in my body.
13. I am choosing whole foods that fuel me.
14. I am moving my body in ways that bring me joy.
15. I am staying hydrated throughout the day.
16. I am walking outside daily and feeling my mood lift.
17. I am enjoying steady energy without the 3pm crash.
18. I am caring for my skin and feeling radiant.
19. I am sleeping deeply and waking refreshed.
20. I am celebrating small health wins with pride.

Parenting with Presence

21. I am listening to my child with full attention.

22. I am creating meaningful family rituals.

23. I am responding calmly in stressful moments.

24. I am patient and present in my child's learning.

25. I am modelling rest and reset for my children.

26. I am enjoying unrushed family meals.

27. I am laughing and playing with my children daily.

28. I am setting boundaries with confidence and love.

29. I am supporting my child's unique personality.

30. I am creating special one-to-one moments with each child.

Home & Daily Flow

31. I am moving through smooth, calm mornings.

32. I am keeping on top of laundry with ease.

33. I am enjoying a lighter home with less clutter.

34. I am resetting my week with a Sunday routine.

35. I am meal-planning with simplicity.

36. I am using a family calendar that works for us.

37. I am teaching my children to help with chores.

38. I am living in a peaceful, welcoming home.

39. I am creating beauty in my space each day.

40. I am choosing rest over chores without guilt.

Identity & Joy Rediscovered

41. I am reconnecting with my hobbies and passions.

42. I am reading books that inspire and delight me.

43. I am enjoying regular girls' nights out.

44. I am treating myself to solo coffee or nature dates.

45. I am planning and booking exciting experiences.

46. I am smiling at my vision board each day.

47. I am comfortable and confident in my own skin.

48. I am filling my week with what lights me up.

49. I am having meaningful, uplifting conversations.

50. I am thriving, not just surviving.

Appendix 2 - Brain Blocks: The Stressful Thoughts Holding You Back

Time & Productivity

1. I never have enough time.
2. I'm always behind.
3. I can't keep up with everything.
4. I waste so much time.
5. I should be more organised.
6. I'm always late.
7. I'll never get on top of my to-do list.
8. I'm not productive enough.
9. I can't focus on anything properly.
10. I'm terrible at managing time.

Health & Body

11. I should be thinner by now.
12. I've let myself go.
13. I'm too tired to exercise.
14. I'll never lose this baby weight.
15. I don't look after myself properly.
16. My body is broken.
17. I look old compared to other mums.
18. I don't deserve to rest until everything else is done.
19. I can't control my eating.
20. I should have more energy.

Parenting & Family

21. I'm not a good enough mum.
22. I lose my temper too often.
23. My kids deserve better.
24. I should spend more quality time with them.
25. I'm messing my kids up.
26. I'm too distracted.
27. I shout too much.
28. I don't have the patience I should.
29. I should enjoy motherhood more.
30. Other mums are doing it better.

Home & Responsibilities

31. My house is always a mess.
32. I can't stay on top of laundry.
33. I'm a bad wife/partner because I don't keep up.
34. I should be more organised with meals.
35. Everyone else has a nicer home.
36. I'm not disciplined enough.
37. I'll never get my house in order.
38. I'm always letting someone down.
39. I'm failing at keeping everything together.
40. I can't do it all.

Identity & Self-Worth

41. I've lost myself.

42. I don't know who I am anymore.

43. I'm just "mum" now.

44. I'm not interesting.

45. I've wasted my potential.

46. I should be further ahead in life.

47. I'm not as successful as my friends.

48. I'm too old to change.

49. I'm not smart enough.

50. I'm not strong enough.

Relationships & Comparison

51. My marriage isn't as good as it should be.

52. I don't give my partner enough attention.

53. We don't connect anymore.

54. I'm letting everyone down.

55. My friends are doing better than me.

56. I'm boring compared to other women.

57. Nobody understands me.

58. I'm too moody to be around.

59. People must think I'm lazy.

60. I'm not fun anymore.

Work & Money

61. I should be earning more.

62. I'm not contributing enough financially.

63. I don't have a proper career anymore.

64. I've wasted my education.

65. I can't juggle work and family.

66. I'm always behind at work.

67. I'm not good at my job.

68. I'll never catch up.

69. I should be further ahead by now.

70. I'm not disciplined with money.

Guilt & Pressure

71. I feel guilty no matter what I do.

72. I'm always failing someone.

73. I should be able to do it all.

74. I never do enough.

75. I'll never get it right.

Appendix 3- Emotions and Where They Show Up in the Body

Overwhelm – heavy chest, tight shoulders, racing heart.

Guilt – sinking stomach, heaviness in the chest.

Frustration – clenched jaw, tense fists, heat in the face.

Exhaustion – drooping eyelids, heavy limbs, aching back.

Anxiety – fluttering stomach, shaky hands, shallow breathing.

Resentment – tight throat, clenched jaw, burning in the chest.

Loneliness – aching chest, hollow stomach, low energy.

Hopelessness – slumped posture, heavy chest, weak legs.

Shame – flushed face, hunched shoulders, knot in the stomach.

Fear – cold hands, pounding heart, butterflies in stomach.

Sadness – lump in throat, watery eyes, heaviness in the chest.

Stress – tight neck, tense shoulders, shallow breath.

Anger – clenched teeth, hot face, fast heartbeat.

Irritation – twitchy fingers, tapping feet, stiff jaw.

Worry – frown lines, tight stomach, racing thoughts.

Inadequacy – sinking posture, weak chest, churning gut.

Confusion – pressure in the head, furrowed brow, restless legs.

Self-doubt – cold hands, hollow chest, tense stomach.

Impatience – tapping feet, restless legs, shallow breathing.

Helplessness – weak knees, slumped back, low energy.

Embarrassment – flushed cheeks, sweating, shaky voice.

Regret – heavy heart, pit in the stomach, restless hands.

Jealousy – tight jaw, burning chest, tense shoulders.

Disappointment – sagging shoulders, dull eyes, empty stomach.

Isolation – ache in chest, lump in throat, tired body.

Stressful anticipation – racing heart, jittery legs, shallow breath.

Conflicted – knot in the stomach, tense chest, restless hands.

Insecurity – hunched shoulders, shallow breath, churning gut.

Pressure – pounding head, stiff neck, tense back.

Hopeless longing – aching heart, faraway eyes, heavy sighs.

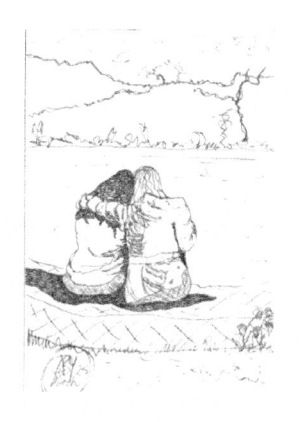

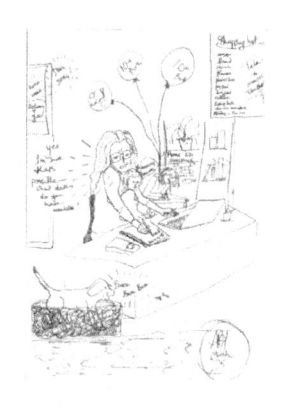

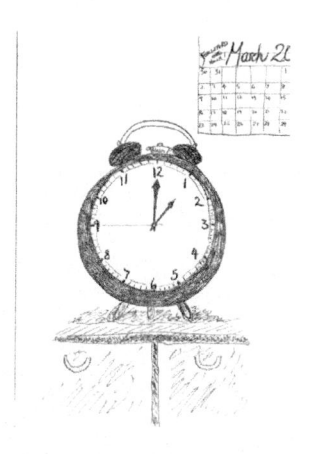

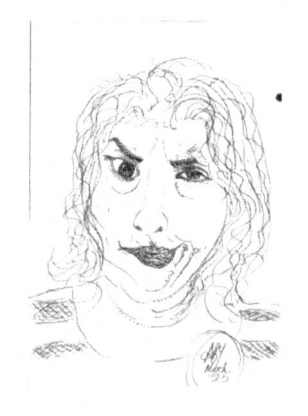

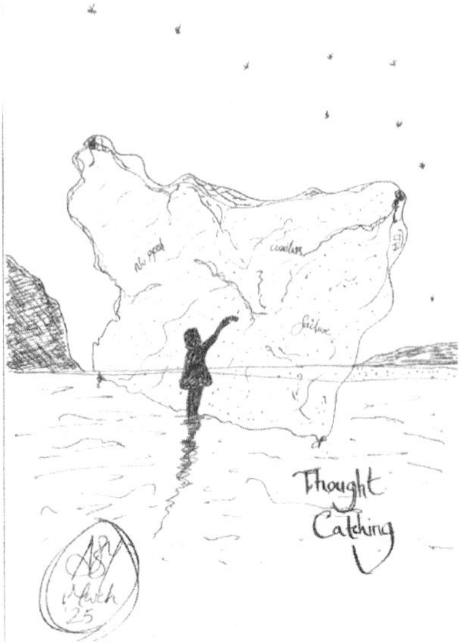
Thought
Catching

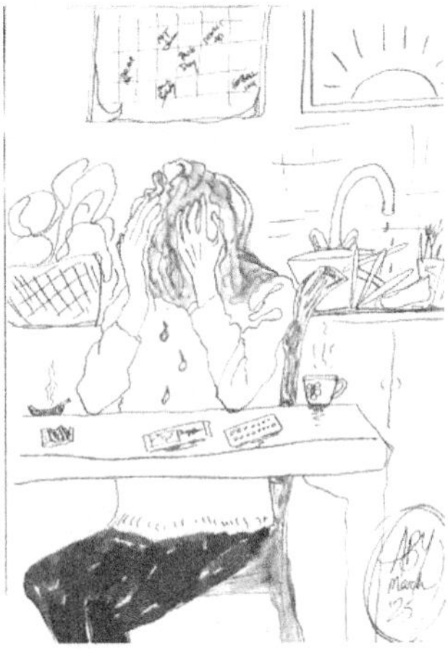

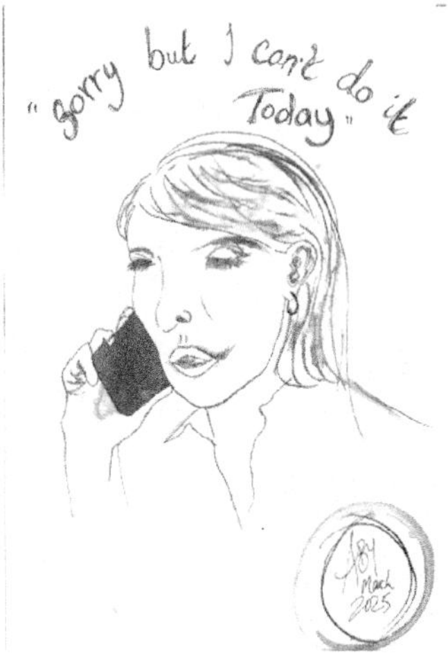
"sorry but I can't do it Today"

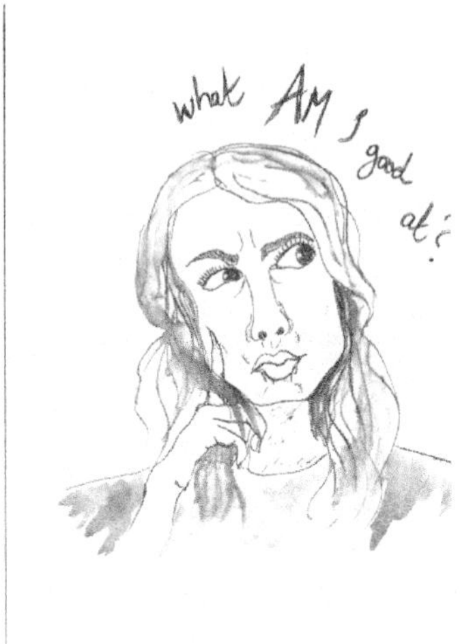
what AM I good at?

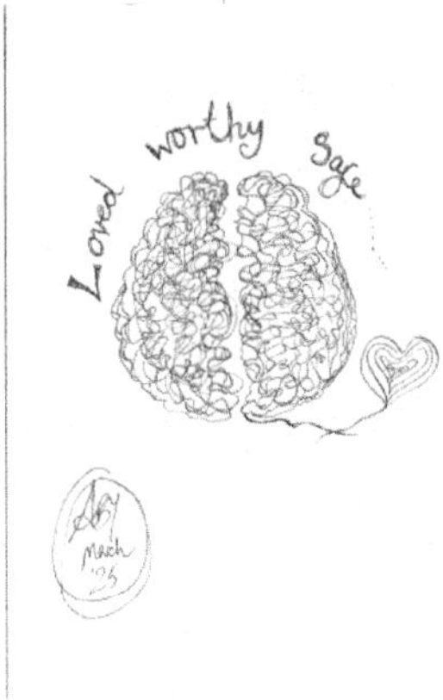
Loved worthy Safe

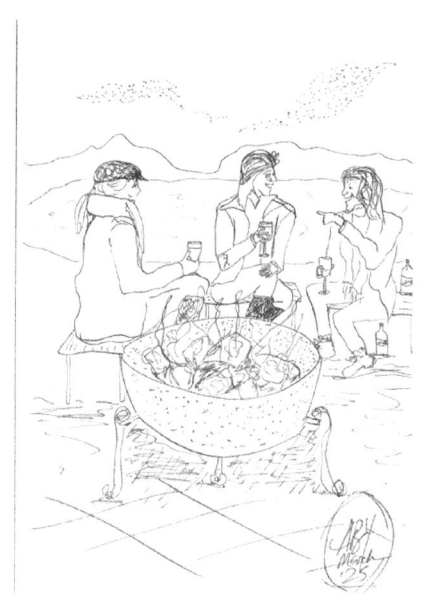

Contact Information

Social media @thedevonshireshepherdess

Website www.thedevonshireshepherdess.co.uk

Email leanne@thedevonshireshepherdess.co.uk

Whats App:

Printed in Dunstable, United Kingdom